2015 Handbook of
EMERGENCY
CARDIOVASCULAR CARE
for Healthcare Providers

With materials adapted from

2015 AHA Guidelines Update for CPR and ECC
2010 AHA Guidelines for CPR and ECC
Basic Life Support
Pediatric Advanced Life Support
Neonatal Resuscitation Textbook
Advanced Cardiovascular Life Support
AHA/ACC Guidelines for Management of STEMI
    and NSTE-ACS

Acknowledgments

The American Heart Association thanks the following people for their contributions to the development of this handbook: Mary Fran Hazinski, RN, MSN; Michael Shuster, MD; Michael W. Donnino, MD; Steven M. Schexnayder, MD; Ricardo A. Samson, MD; Andrew H. Travers, MD, MSc; Sallie Young, PharmD, BCPS; Myra H. Wyckoff, MD; Venu Menon, MD; Peter D. Panagos, MD; Eric J. Lavonas, MD; and the AHA ECC Handbook Project Team.

i

Contents

Pediatric Advanced Life Support

Preface

This 2015 edition of the *Handbook of Emergency Cardiovascular Care for Healthcare Providers* includes the latest algorithms and reference material from the *2015 AHA Guidelines Update for CPR and ECC,* integrated with content from the *2010 AHA Guidelines for CPR and ECC.*

The integrated *2015 AHA Guidelines for CPR and ECC,* available at **ECCguidelines.heart.org** represents the best current understanding of science and translation of the science into direct patient care. It is based on the *2015 International Consensus on CPR and ECC Science With Treatment Recommendations.* This international review is now continuous and can be found at **www.ilcor.org/seers**.

The material in this handbook was selected for its relevance to patient care and its application to a quick-reference format. While these recommendations are based in an extensive international science review, not all recommendations will apply to all rescuers and all victims in all situations. The leader of any resuscitation must be prepared to adapt these recommendations to patient needs and circumstances.

The *2015 AHA Guidelines Update for CPR and ECC* marks the 55th year since the publication of the landmark article by Kouwenhoven, Jude, and Knickerbocker reporting increased survival from cardiac arrest with focus on providing high-quality CPR and post–cardiac arrest support. With such efforts, as well as a continued commitment to the advancement of resuscitation science, thousands of lives can be saved every year.

Mary Fran Hazinski
Michael Shuster

Note on Medication Doses

Emergency cardiovascular care is a dynamic science. Advances in treatment and drug therapies occur rapidly. Readers are advised to check for changes in recommended dose, indications, and contraindications in future editions of this handbook and AHA training materials, as well as the package insert product information sheet for each drug.

Clinical condition and pharmacokinetics may require drug dose or interval dosing adjustments. Specific parameters may require monitoring, for example, of creatinine clearance or QT interval. Some medications listed in this handbook may not be available in all countries, and may not be specifically approved by regulatory agencies in some countries for a particular indication.

Copyright Notice

To find out about any updates or corrections to this text, visit **www.heart.org/cpr**, navigate to the page for this product, and click on "Updates."

Recognition and Activation/CPR and Rescue Breathing/Defibrillation

The following sequence is intended for a single healthcare provider rescuer. If additional rescuers are available, the first rescuer feels for a pulse for no more than 10 seconds and starts chest compressions if the pulse is not definitely palpated. A second rescuer activates the emergency response number and obtains an automated external defibrillator (AED), and a third rescuer opens the airway and provides ventilation. If additional trained rescuers are available, they will perform many steps simultaneously.

For patients with known or suspected opioid overdose, refer to the Opioid-Associated Life-Threatening Emergency (Adult) Algorithm.

Recognition
The victim is not responsive and not breathing or only gasping (ie, not breathing normally). Trained rescuers are encouraged to simultaneously perform some steps (ie, checking for breathing and pulse at the same time) in an effort to reduce time to first compressions and defibrillation.

Activation
Activate the emergency response system or resuscitation team after finding the victim unresponsive or after identifying respiratory or cardiac arrest, as appropriate to clinical setting or protocol. Retrieve or send someone to retrieve the AED and emergency equipment.

Pulse Check
Check for a pulse for no more than 10 seconds (carotid in adult; carotid or femoral in child; brachial in infant).

- *If pulse absent:* Provide CPR (start with chest compressions and perform cycles of 30 compressions and 2 breaths) until an AED or advanced life support (ALS) providers arrive. For 2 rescuers, the compression-ventilation ratio for infants and children (to the age of puberty) is 15:2.

- *If pulse present* but breathing is absent: Open the airway and provide rescue breathing (1 breath every 5 to 6 seconds for adult; 1 breath every 3 to 5 seconds for infant or child). Recheck the pulse about every 2 minutes.

- *In infant or child with adequate oxygenation and ventilation if pulse present but ≤60/min with poor perfusion:* Begin chest compressions with ventilations.

CPR (C-A-B)

C. Compressions
Begin CPR with 30 chest compressions. (If 2 rescuers for infant or child, provide 15 compressions.)

A. Open airway
After chest compressions, open the airway with a head tilt–chin lift or jaw thrust.

B. Breathing
Give 2 breaths that make the chest rise. Release completely; allow for exhalation between breaths. After 2 breaths, immediately resume chest compressions. Give each breath over 1 second.

Continue Basic Life Support Until Advanced Providers Arrive
Continue CPR until ALS providers take over or the victim starts to move. Integrate newborn resuscitation, pediatric advanced life support, or advanced cardiovascular life support at the earliest opportunity.

Defibrillation
Attach and use an AED as soon as it is available. Minimize interruptions in chest compressions before and after shock. If no shock is needed, and after any shock delivery, immediately resume CPR, starting with chest compressions.

Component	Adults and Adolescents	Children (Age 1 Year to Puberty)	Infants (Age Less Than 1 Year, Excluding Newborns)
Scene safety	Make sure the environment is safe for rescuers and victim		
Recognition of cardiac arrest	Check for responsiveness No breathing or only gasping (ie, no normal breathing) No definite pulse felt within 10 seconds (Breathing and pulse check can be performed simultaneously in less than 10 seconds)		
Activation of emergency response system	If you are alone with no mobile phone, leave the victim to activate the emergency response system and get the AED before beginning CPR Otherwise, send someone and begin CPR immediately; use the AED as soon as it is available	*Witnessed collapse* Follow steps for adults and adolescents on the left *Unwitnessed collapse* Give 2 minutes of CPR Leave the victim to activate the emergency response system and get the AED Return to the child or infant and resume CPR; use the AED as soon as it is available	
Compression-ventilation ratio *without advanced airway*	*1 or 2 rescuers* 30:2	*1 rescuer* 30:2 *2 or more rescuers* 15:2	

Compression-ventilation ratio *with advanced airway*	Continuous compressions at a rate of 100-120/min Give 1 breath every 6 seconds (10 breaths/min)		
Compression rate	100-120/min		
Compression depth	At least 2 inches (5 cm)*	At least one third AP diameter of chest About 2 inches (5 cm)	At least one third AP diameter of chest About 1½ inches (4 cm)
Hand placement	2 hands on the lower half of the breastbone (sternum)	2 hands or 1 hand (optional for very small child) on the lower half of the breastbone (sternum)	*1 rescuer* 2 fingers in the center of the chest, just below the nipple line *2 or more rescuers* 2 thumb–encircling hands in the center of the chest, just below the nipple line
Chest recoil	Allow full recoil of chest after each compression; do not lean on the chest after each compression		
Minimizing interruptions	Limit interruptions in chest compressions to less than 10 seconds		

*Compression depth should be no more than 2.4 inches (6 cm).

Abbreviations: AED, automated external defibrillator; AP, anteroposterior; CPR, cardiopulmonary resuscitation.

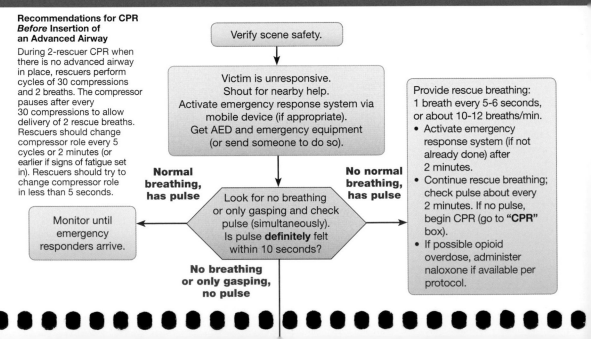

Recommendations for CPR *Before* Insertion of an Advanced Airway

During 2-rescuer CPR when there is no advanced airway in place, rescuers perform cycles of 30 compressions and 2 breaths. The compressor pauses after every 30 compressions to allow delivery of 2 rescue breaths. Rescuers should change compressor role every 5 cycles or 2 minutes (or earlier if signs of fatigue set in). Rescuers should try to change compressor role in less than 5 seconds.

Verify scene safety.

Victim is unresponsive.
Shout for nearby help.
Activate emergency response system via mobile device (if appropriate).
Get AED and emergency equipment (or send someone to do so).

Normal breathing, has pulse

Monitor until emergency responders arrive.

Look for no breathing or only gasping and check pulse (simultaneously). Is pulse **definitely** felt within 10 seconds?

No breathing or only gasping, no pulse

No normal breathing, has pulse

Provide rescue breathing:
1 breath every 5-6 seconds, or about 10-12 breaths/min.
- Activate emergency response system (if not already done) after 2 minutes.
- Continue rescue breathing; check pulse about every 2 minutes. If no pulse, begin CPR (go to **"CPR"** box).
- If possible opioid overdose, administer naloxone if available per protocol.

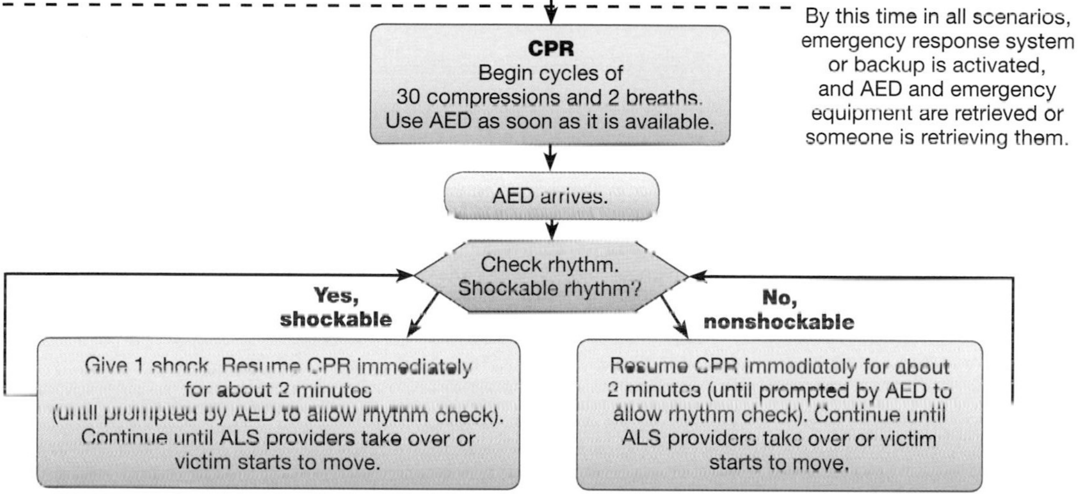

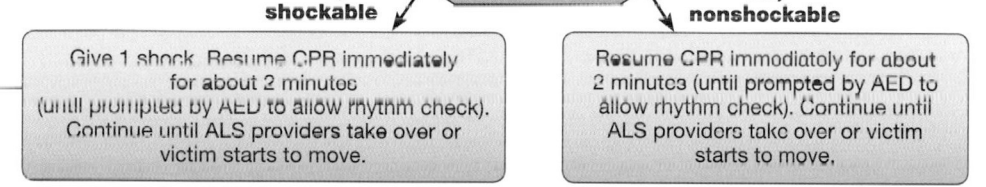

CPR
Begin cycles of
30 compressions and 2 breaths.
Use AED as soon as it is available.

By this time in all scenarios,
emergency response system
or backup is activated,
and AED and emergency
equipment are retrieved or
someone is retrieving them.

AED arrives.

Check rhythm.
Shockable rhythm?

Yes, shockable

Give 1 shock. Resume CPR immediately
for about 2 minutes
(until prompted by AED to allow rhythm check).
Continue until ALS providers take over or
victim starts to move.

No, nonshockable

Resume CPR immediately for about
2 minutes (until prompted by AED to
allow rhythm check). Continue until
ALS providers take over or victim
starts to move.

Recommendations for CPR *After* Insertion of an Advanced Airway

Once an advanced airway is in place, 2 rescuers no longer deliver "cycles" of CPR (compressions interrupted by pauses for ventilation). Instead, the compressing rescuer should give continuous chest compressions at a rate of 100-120/min without pauses for ventilation. The rescuer delivering ventilation provides 1 breath every 6 seconds (10 breaths/min). Two or more rescuers should change compressor role approximately every 2 minutes (or earlier if signs of fatigue set in) to prevent compressor fatigue and deterioration in quality and rate of chest compressions given. Rescuers should try to change compressor role in less than 5 seconds.

Relief of Foreign-Body Airway Obstruction

Adults and Adolescents	Children (Age 1 Year to Puberty)	Infants (Age Less Than 1 Year)
1. Ask "Are you choking?" If the victim nods "yes" and cannot talk, severe airway obstruction is present. Take steps immediately to relieve the obstruction.	1. Ask "Are you choking?" If the victim nods "yes" and cannot talk, severe airway obstruction is present. Take steps immediately to relieve the obstruction.	1. If the victim cannot make any sounds or breathe, severe airway obstruction is present.
2. Give abdominal thrusts/Heimlich maneuver or chest thrusts for pregnant or obese victims.	2. Give abdominal thrusts/Heimlich maneuver.	2. Give up to 5 back slaps *and* up to 5 chest thrusts.
3. Repeat abdominal thrusts (or chest thrusts if the victim is pregnant or obese) until effective or the victim becomes unresponsive.	3. Repeat abdominal thrusts until effective or the victim becomes unresponsive.	3. Repeat step 2 until effective or the victim becomes unresponsive.

Victim becomes unresponsive

4. Activate the emergency response system via mobile device (if appropriate) or send someone to do so. After about 2 minutes of CPR, if you are alone with no mobile device, leave the victim to activate the emergency response system (if no one has already done so).
5. Lower the victim to the floor. Begin CPR, starting with chest compressions. Do not check for a pulse.
6. Before you deliver breaths, look into the mouth. If you see a foreign body that can be easily removed, remove it.
7. Continue CPR until advanced providers arrive.

Refer to Basic Life Support course materials for more information about relief of foreign-body airway obstruction.

BLS Dos and Don'ts of Adult High-Quality CPR

Rescuers Should	Rescuers Should *Not*
Perform chest compressions at a rate of 100-120/min	Compress at a rate slower than 100/min or faster than 120/min
Compress to a depth of at least 2 inches (5 cm)	Compress at a depth of less than 2 inches (5 cm) or greater than 2.4 inches (6 cm)
Allow full recoil after each compression	Lean on the chest between compressions
Minimize pauses in compressions	Interrupt compressions for greater than 10 seconds
Ventilate adequately (2 breaths after 30 compressions, each breath delivered over 1 second, each causing chest rise)	Provide excessive ventilation (ie, too many breaths or breaths with excessive force)

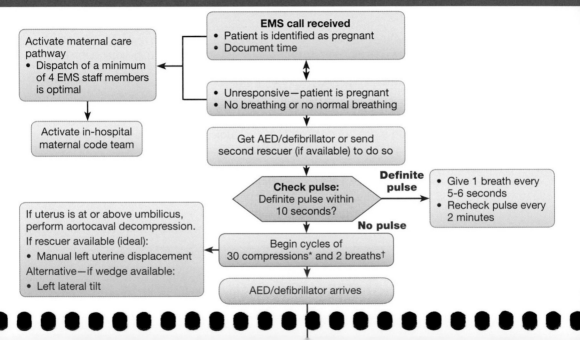

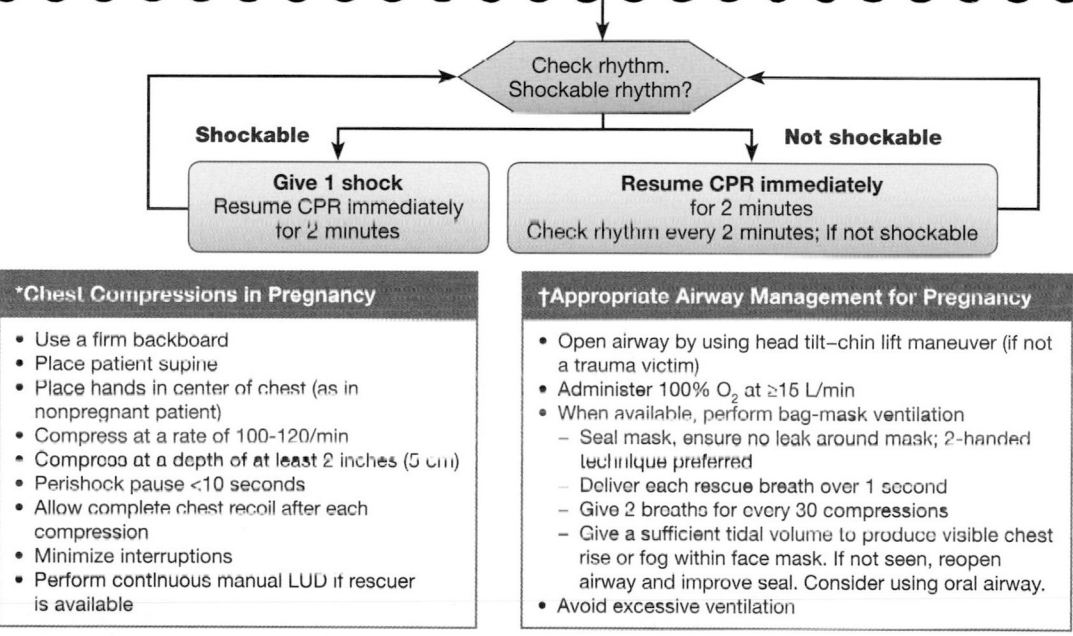

```
                    Check rhythm.
                    Shockable rhythm?
```

Shockable — **Not shockable**

Give 1 shock
Resume CPR immediately
for 2 minutes

Resume CPR immediately
for 2 minutes
Check rhythm every 2 minutes; If not shockable

*Chest Compressions in Pregnancy

- Use a firm backboard
- Place patient supine
- Place hands in center of chest (as in nonpregnant patient)
- Compress at a rate of 100-120/min
- Compress at a depth of at least 2 inches (5 cm)
- Perishock pause <10 seconds
- Allow complete chest recoil after each compression
- Minimize interruptions
- Perform continuous manual LUD if rescuer is available

†Appropriate Airway Management for Pregnancy

- Open airway by using head tilt–chin lift maneuver (if not a trauma victim)
- Administer 100% O_2 at ≥15 L/min
- When available, perform bag-mask ventilation
  - Seal mask, ensure no leak around mask; 2-handed technique preferred
  - Deliver each rescue breath over 1 second
  - Give 2 breaths for every 30 compressions
  - Give a sufficient tidal volume to produce visible chest rise or fog within face mask. If not seen, reopen airway and improve seal. Consider using oral airway.
- Avoid excessive ventilation

Cardiac Arrest in Pregnancy In-Hospital BLS Algorithm: Simultaneous C-A-B-U—New 2015

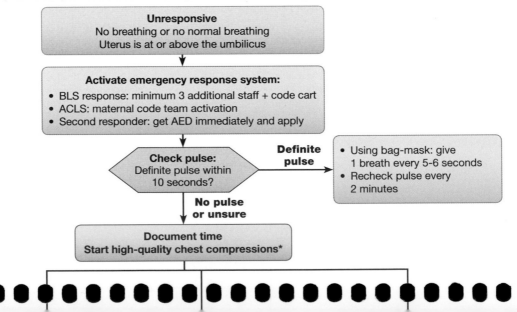

(**C**hest compressions/**C**urrent-**A**irway-**B**reathing-**U**terine displacement)

Unresponsive
No breathing or no normal breathing
Uterus is at or above the umbilicus

Activate emergency response system:
- BLS response: minimum 3 additional staff + code cart
- ACLS: maternal code team activation
- Second responder: get AED immediately and apply

Check pulse:
Definite pulse within
10 seconds?

Definite pulse
- Using bag-mask: give 1 breath every 5-6 seconds
- Recheck pulse every 2 minutes

No pulse or unsure

Document time
Start high-quality chest compressions*

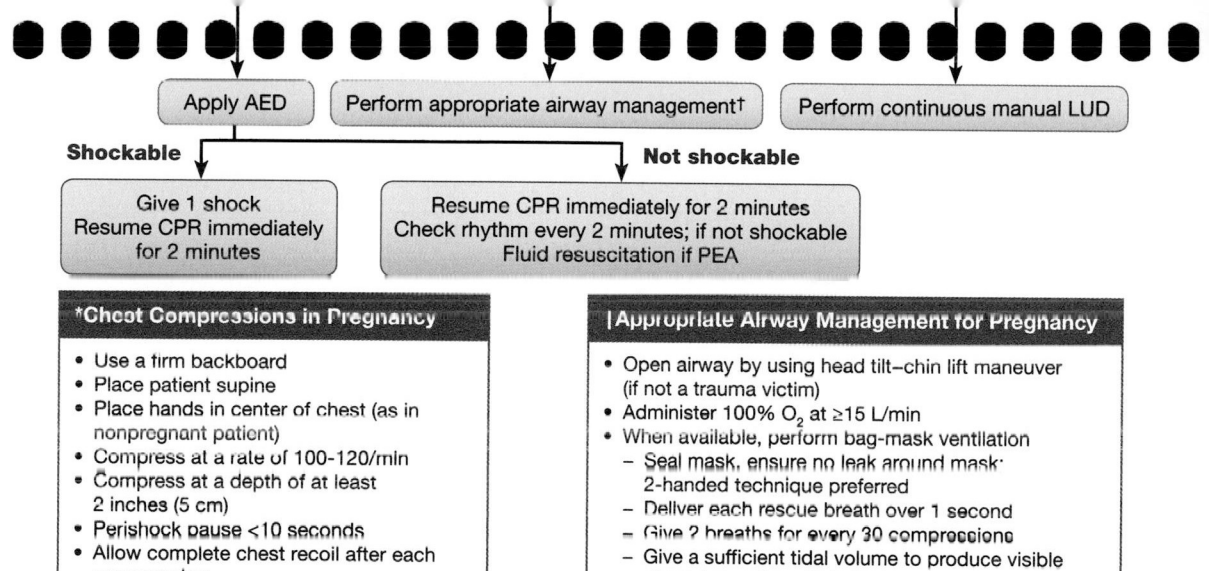

Apply AED | **Perform appropriate airway management†** | **Perform continuous manual LUD**

Shockable

Give 1 shock
Resume CPR immediately
for 2 minutes

Not shockable

Resume CPR immediately for 2 minutes
Check rhythm every 2 minutes; if not shockable
Fluid resuscitation if PEA

*Chest Compressions in Pregnancy

- Use a firm backboard
- Place patient supine
- Place hands in center of chest (as in nonpregnant patient)
- Compress at a rate of 100-120/min
- Compress at a depth of at least 2 inches (5 cm)
- Perishock pause <10 seconds
- Allow complete chest recoil after each compression
- Minimize interruptions
- Perform continuous manual LUD

|Appropriate Airway Management for Pregnancy

- Open airway by using head tilt–chin lift maneuver (if not a trauma victim)
- Administer 100% O_2 at ≥15 L/min
- When available, perform bag-mask ventilation
  - Seal mask, ensure no leak around mask; 2-handed technique preferred
  - Deliver each rescue breath over 1 second
  - Give 2 breaths for every 30 compressions
  - Give a sufficient tidal volume to produce visible chest rise or fog within face mask. If not seen, reopen airway and improve seal. Consider using oral airway.
- Avoid excessive ventilation

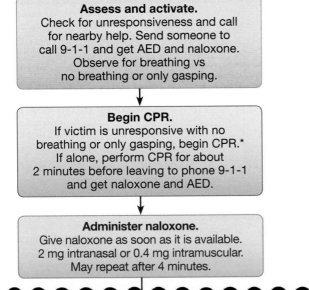

Assess and activate.
Check for unresponsiveness and call for nearby help. Send someone to call 9-1-1 and get AED and naloxone. Observe for breathing vs no breathing or only gasping.

Begin CPR.
If victim is unresponsive with no breathing or only gasping, begin CPR.*
If alone, perform CPR for about 2 minutes before leaving to phone 9-1-1 and get naloxone and AED.

Administer naloxone.
Give naloxone as soon as it is available. 2 mg intranasal or 0.4 mg intramuscular. May repeat after 4 minutes.

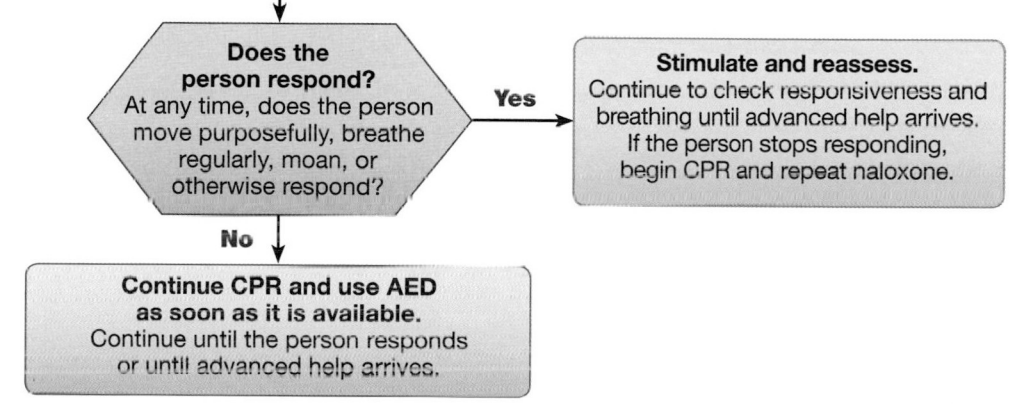

Does the person respond?
At any time, does the person move purposefully, breathe regularly, moan, or otherwise respond?

Yes →

Stimulate and reassess.
Continue to check responsiveness and breathing until advanced help arrives. If the person stops responding, begin CPR and repeat naloxone.

No ↓

Continue CPR and use AED as soon as it is available.
Continue until the person responds or until advanced help arrives.

*CPR technique based on rescuer's level of training.

Team-Based Resuscitation

ACLS

The team owns the code. No team member leaves the triangle except to protect his or her safety.

Resuscitation Triangle Roles

Compressor

- Assesses the patient
- Does 5 cycles of chest compressions
- Alternates with AED/Monitor/ Defibrillator every 5 cycles or 2 minutes (or earlier if signs of fatigue set in)

AED/Monitor/ Defibrillator

- Brings and operates the AED/monitor/defibrillator
- Alternates with Compressor every 5 cycles or 2 minutes (or earlier if signs of fatigue set in), ideally during rhythm analysis
- If a monitor is present, places it in a position where it can be seen by the Team Leader (and most of the team)

Airway

- Opens the airway
- Provides bag-mask ventilation
- Inserts airway adjuncts as appropriate

Positions for 6-Person High-Performance Teams*

*This is a suggested team formation. Roles may be adapted to local protocol.

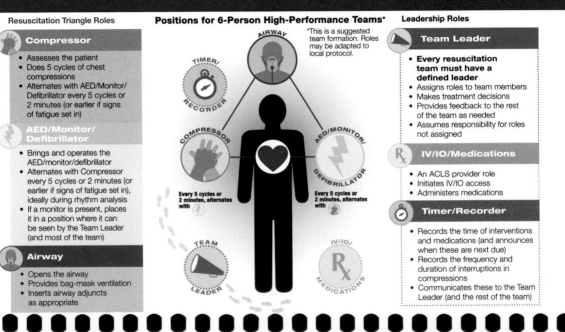

Every 5 cycles or 2 minutes, alternates with

Every 5 cycles or 2 minutes, alternates with

Leadership Roles

Team Leader

- **Every resuscitation team must have a defined leader**
- Assigns roles to team members
- Makes treatment decisions
- Provides feedback to the rest of the team as needed
- Assumes responsibility for roles not assigned

IV/IO/Medications

- An ACLS provider role
- Initiates IV/IO access
- Administers medications

Timer/Recorder

- Records the time of interventions and medications (and announces when these are next due)
- Records the frequency and duration of interruptions in compressions
- Communicates these to the Team Leader (and the rest of the team)

Priority-Based Multiple-Rescuer Response

This figure illustrates a potential seamless, time-sensitive, integrated team-based approach to resuscitation where roles and interventions are prioritized and distributed as more resources arrive to the patient.

Times (in seconds) may vary based on circumstances, response times, and local protocols.

*With 2 or more rescuers, one healthcare provider (HCP) should assume the role of Team Leader.

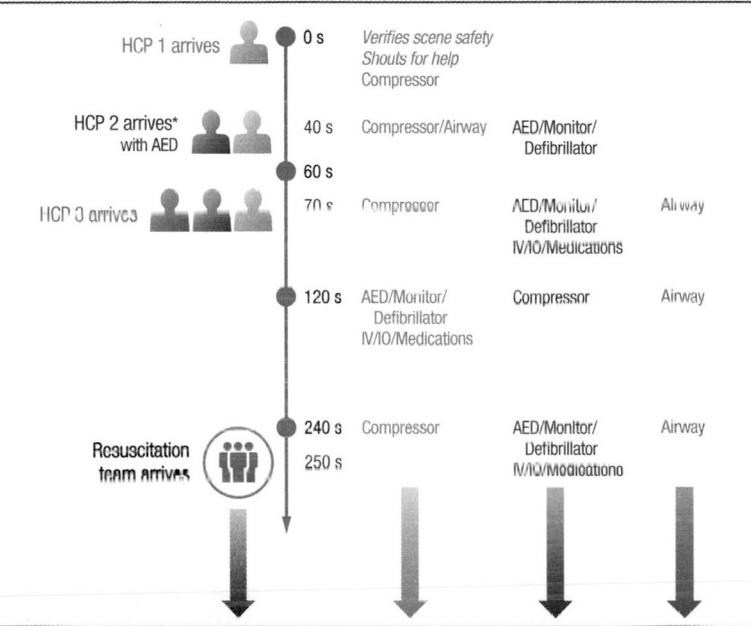

HCP 1 arrives	0 s	Verifies scene safety / Shouts for help / Compressor	
HCP 2 arrives* with AED	40 s	Compressor/Airway	AED/Monitor/Defibrillator
	60 s		
HCP 3 arrives	70 s	Compressor	AED/Monitor/Defibrillator / IV/IO/Medications	Airway
	120 s	AED/Monitor/Defibrillator / IV/IO/Medications	Compressor	Airway
Resuscitation team arrives	240 s / 250 s	Compressor	AED/Monitor/Defibrillator / IV/IO/Medications	Airway

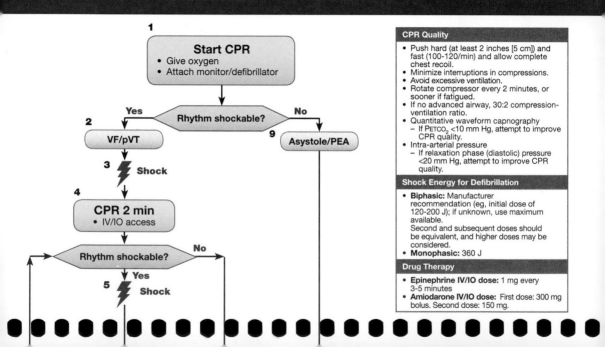

1

Start CPR
- Give oxygen
- Attach monitor/defibrillator

Yes — Rhythm shockable? — **No**

2 VF/pVT

9 Asystole/PEA

3 Shock

4

CPR 2 min
- IV/IO access

Rhythm shockable? — **No**

Yes

5 Shock

CPR Quality

- Push hard (at least 2 inches [5 cm]) and fast (100-120/min) and allow complete chest recoil.
- Minimize interruptions in compressions.
- Avoid excessive ventilation.
- Rotate compressor every 2 minutes, or sooner if fatigued.
- If no advanced airway, 30:2 compression-ventilation ratio.
- Quantitative waveform capnography
  - If P_{ETCO_2} <10 mm Hg, attempt to improve CPR quality.
- Intra-arterial pressure
  - If relaxation phase (diastolic) pressure <20 mm Hg, attempt to improve CPR quality.

Shock Energy for Defibrillation

- **Biphasic:** Manufacturer recommendation (eg, initial dose of 120-200 J); if unknown, use maximum available.
  Second and subsequent doses should be equivalent, and higher doses may be considered.
- **Monophasic:** 360 J

Drug Therapy

- **Epinephrine IV/IO dose:** 1 mg every 3-5 minutes
- **Amiodarone IV/IO dose:** First dose: 300 mg bolus. Second dose: 150 mg.

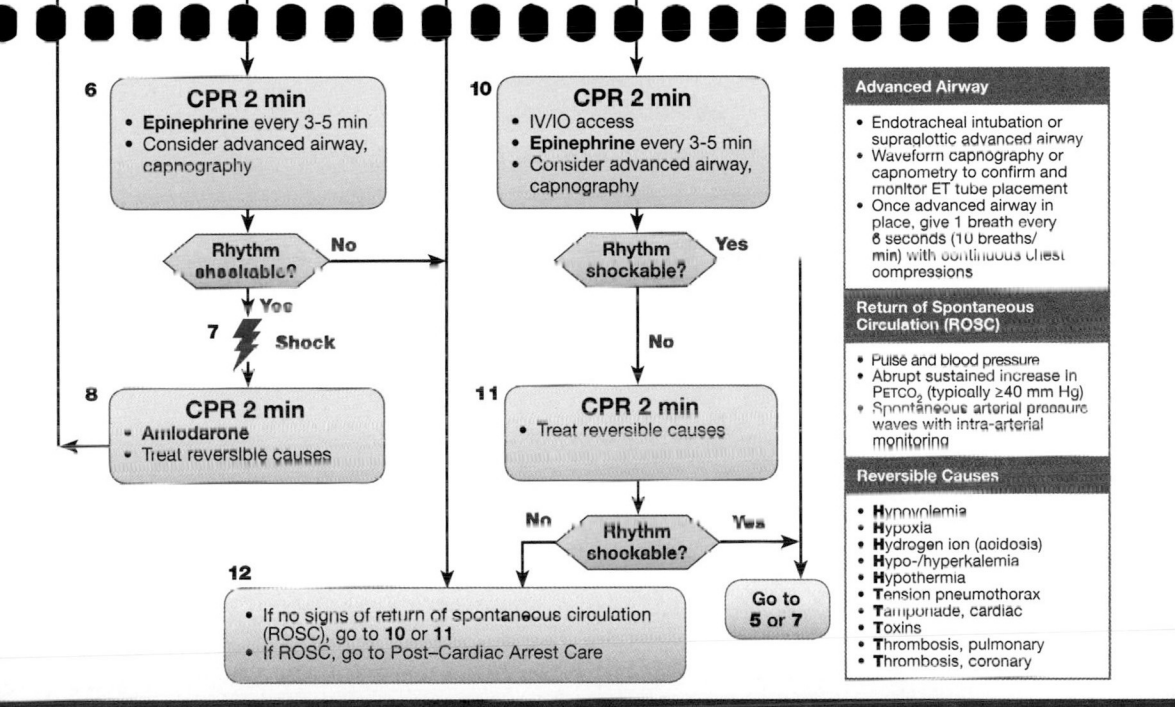

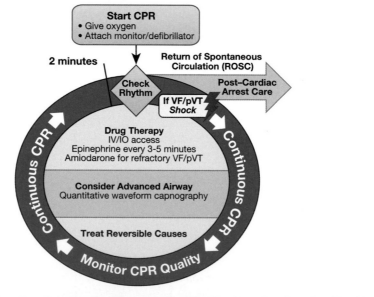

CPR Quality

- Push hard (at least 2 inches [5 cm]) and fast (100-120/min) and allow complete chest recoil.
- Minimize interruptions in compressions.
- Avoid excessive ventilation.
- Rotate compressor every 2 minutes, or sooner if fatigued.
- If no advanced airway, 30:2 compression-ventilation ratio.
- Quantitative waveform capnography
  – If $PETCO_2$ <10 mm Hg, attempt to improve CPR quality.
- Intra-arterial pressure
  – If relaxation phase (diastolic) pressure <20 mm Hg, attempt to improve CPR quality.

Shock Energy for Defibrillation

- **Biphasic:** Manufacturer recommendation (eg, initial dose of 120-200 J); if unknown, use maximum available. Second and subsequent doses should be equivalent, and higher doses may be considered.
- **Monophasic:** 360 J

Drug Therapy

- **Epinephrine IV/IO dose:** 1 mg every 3-5 minutes
- **Amiodarone IV/IO dose:** First dose: 300 mg bolus. Second dose: 150 mg.

Advanced Airway

- Endotracheal intubation or supraglottic advanced airway
- Waveform capnography or capnometry to confirm and monitor ET tube placement
- Once advanced airway in place, give 1 breath every 6 seconds (10 breaths/min) with continuous chest compressions

Return of Spontaneous Circulation (ROSC)

- Pulse and blood pressure
- Abrupt sustained increase in $PETCO_2$ (typically ≥40 mm Hg)
- Spontaneous arterial pressure waves with intra-arterial monitoring

Reversible Causes

- **H**ypovolemia
- **H**ypoxia
- **H**ydrogen ion (acidosis)
- **H**ypo-/hyperkalemia
- **H**ypothermia
- **T**ension pneumothorax
- **T**amponade, cardiac
- **T**oxins
- **T**hrombosis, pulmonary
- **T**hrombosis, coronary

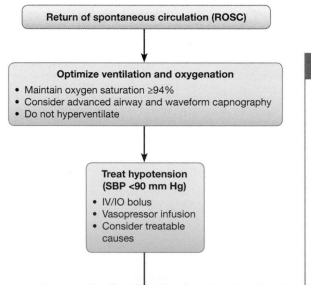

Return of spontaneous circulation (ROSC)

Optimize ventilation and oxygenation

- Maintain oxygen saturation ≥94%
- Consider advanced airway and waveform capnography
- Do not hyperventilate

Treat hypotension (SBP <90 mm Hg)

- IV/IO bolus
- Vasopressor infusion
- Consider treatable causes

Doses/Details

Ventilation/oxygenation:
Avoid excessive ventilation. Start at 10 breaths/min and titrate to target P_{ETCO_2} of 35-40 mm Hg.
When feasible, titrate FIO_2 to minimum necessary to achieve SpO_2 ≥94%.

IV bolus:
Approximately 1-2 L normal saline or lactated Ringer's

Epinephrine IV infusion:
0.1-0.5 mcg/kg per minute (in 70-kg adult: 7-35 mcg per minute)

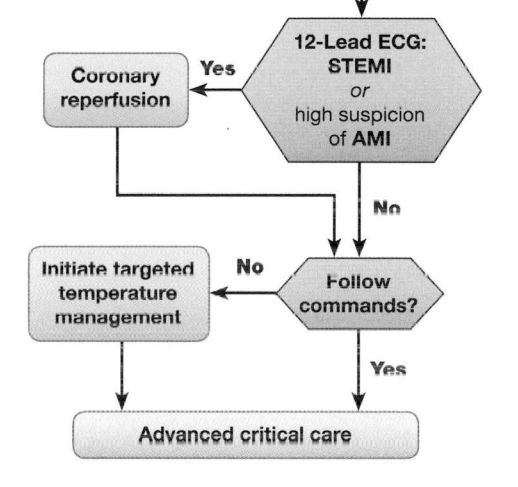

Dopamine IV infusion:
5-10 mcg/kg per minute

**Norepinephrine
IV infusion:**
0.1-0.5 mcg/kg per minute
(in 70-kg adult: 7-35 mcg
per minute)

Reversible Causes

- **H**ypovolemia
- **H**ypoxia
- **H**ydrogen ion (acidosis)
- **H**ypo-/hyperkalemia
- **H**ypothermia
- **T**ension pneumothorax
- **T**amponade, cardiac
- **T**oxins
- **T**hrombosis, pulmonary
- **T**hrombosis, coronary

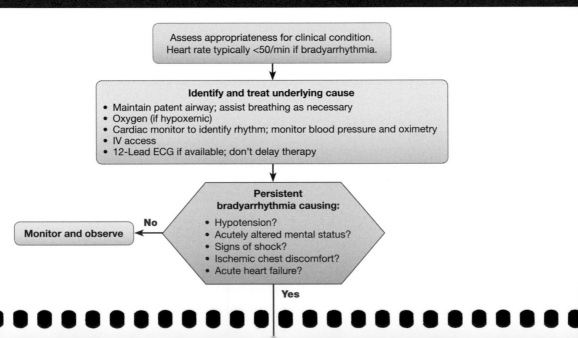

Assess appropriateness for clinical condition.
Heart rate typically <50/min if bradyarrhythmia.

Identify and treat underlying cause

- Maintain patent airway; assist breathing as necessary
- Oxygen (if hypoxemic)
- Cardiac monitor to identify rhythm; monitor blood pressure and oximetry
- IV access
- 12-Lead ECG if available; don't delay therapy

**Persistent
bradyarrhythmia causing:**

- Hypotension?
- Acutely altered mental status?
- Signs of shock?
- Ischemic chest discomfort?
- Acute heart failure?

No

Monitor and observe

Yes

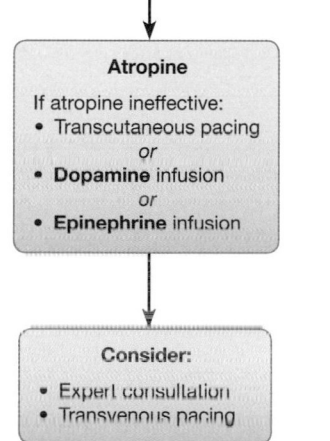

Atropine

If atropine ineffective:
- Transcutaneous pacing
  or
- **Dopamine** infusion
  or
- **Epinephrine** infusion

Consider:
- Expert consultation
- Transvenous pacing

Doses/Details

Atropine IV dose:
First dose: 0.5 mg bolus.
Repeat every 3-5 minutes
Maximum: 3 mg.

Dopamine IV infusion:
Usual infusion rate is
2-20 mcg/kg per minute.
Titrate to patient response;
taper slowly.

Epinephrine IV infusion:
2-10 mcg per minute
infusion. Titrate
to patient response.

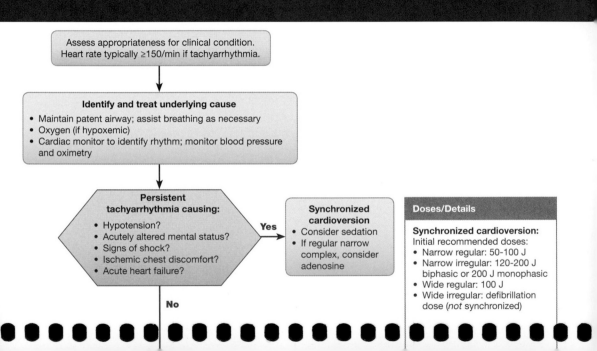

Assess appropriateness for clinical condition.
Heart rate typically ≥150/min if tachyarrhythmia.

Identify and treat underlying cause

- Maintain patent airway; assist breathing as necessary
- Oxygen (if hypoxemic)
- Cardiac monitor to identify rhythm; monitor blood pressure and oximetry

Persistent tachyarrhythmia causing:

- Hypotension?
- Acutely altered mental status?
- Signs of shock?
- Ischemic chest discomfort?
- Acute heart failure?

Yes

No

Synchronized cardioversion

- Consider sedation
- If regular narrow complex, consider adenosine

Doses/Details

Synchronized cardioversion:
Initial recommended doses:

- Narrow regular: 50-100 J
- Narrow irregular: 120-200 J biphasic or 200 J monophasic
- Wide regular: 100 J
- Wide irregular: defibrillation dose (*not* synchronized)

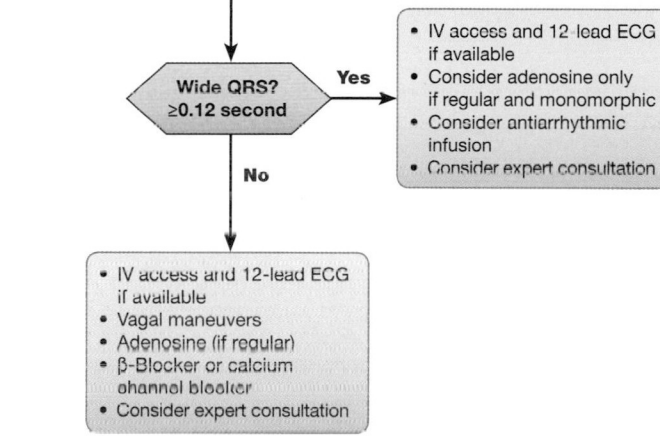

Wide QRS?
≥0.12 second

Yes →
- IV access and 12-lead ECG if available
- Consider adenosine only if regular and monomorphic
- Consider antiarrhythmic infusion
- Consider expert consultation

No ↓
- IV access and 12-lead ECG if available
- Vagal maneuvers
- Adenosine (if regular)
- β-Blocker or calcium channel blocker
- Consider expert consultation

Adenosine IV dose:
First dose: 6 mg rapid IV push; follow with NS flush.
Second dose: 12 mg if required.

Antiarrhythmic Infusions for Stable Wide-QRS Tachycardia

Procainamide IV dose:
20-50 mg/min until arrhythmia suppressed, hypotension ensues, QRS duration increases >50%, or maximum dose 17 mg/kg given Maintenance infusion: 1-4 mg/min.
Avoid if prolonged QT or CHF.

Amiodarone IV dose:
First dose: 150 mg over 10 minutes. Repeat as needed if VT recurs.
Follow by maintenance infusion of 1 mg/min for first 6 hours.

Sotalol IV dose:
100 mg (1.5 mg/kg) over 5 minutes. Avoid if prolonged QT.

Rhythm strips A and B demonstrate the requirement to evaluate the QT interval in light of the heart rate. Strip C depicts an ECG from a patient with a prolonged QT interval.

- *Strip A:* A bradycardic rhythm of 57/min has a QT interval of 0.4 second, which is less than the upper limit of normal for a rate of 57 (0.41 second for a man and 0.45 second for a woman), and a QT/R-R ratio of 38% (<40%).

- *Strip B:* A faster rate of 78/min has a shorter measured QT interval of 0.24 second (faster-shorter/slower-longer), which is less than the upper limit of normal for a rate of 78 (0.35 second for a man and 0.38 second for a woman), and a QT/R-R ratio of 33% (<40%).

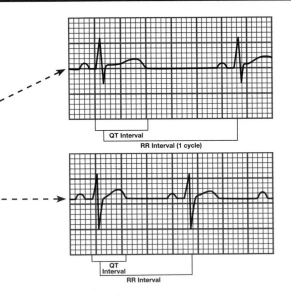

- *Strip C:* Here the QT interval is prolonged at 0.45 second, exceeding the upper limit of normal for a rate of 80/min (0.34 second for a man and 0.37 second for a woman). The QT/R-R ratio of 59% is considerably above the 40% threshold. This strip is from a patient who took an overdose of a tricyclic antidepressant.

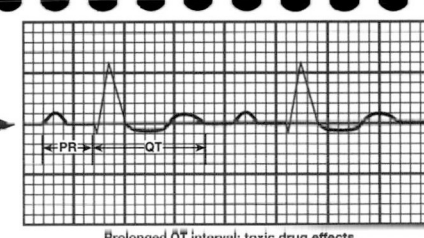

Prolonged QT interval: toxic drug effects

Parameter	Rhythm Strip A	Rhythm Strip B	Rhythm Strip C
Rate	57/min	78/min	80/min
R-R interval (cardiac cycle time)	1.04 seconds (26 × 1-mm boxes)	0.72 second (18 × 1-mm boxes)	0.76 second (19 × 1-mm boxes)
QT interval, measured	0.4 second (10 × 1-mm boxes)	0.24 second (6 × 1-mm boxes)	0.45 second (11 × 1-mm boxes)
QT$_c$ interval: QT interval corrected for heart rate (upper limit of normal QT interval range for a man or a woman from table on next page)	0.41 second (man) 0.45 second (woman)	0.35 second (man) 0.39 second (woman)	0.34 second (man) 0.37 second (woman)
QT/R-R ratio: QT interval divided by R-R interval	38% (0.4/1.04 = 0.384)	33% (0.24/0.72 = 0.333)	59% (0.45/0.76 = 0.592)

From Cummins RO, Graves JR. *ACLS Scenarios: Core Concepts for Case-Based Learning.* St Louis, MO: Mosby Lifeline; 1996. Figures modified with permission from Elsevier.

Maximum QT Interval (Upper Limits of Normal) for Men and Women Based on Heart Rate

Note the relationship between decreasing heart rate and increasing maximum QT interval. For normal heart range of 60 to 100 per minute (gray), the maximum QT intervals for men and women (light blue) are less than one half the R-R interval (green). Most people estimate QT and R-R intervals by counting the number of 1-mm boxes and then multiplying by 0.04 second.

Heart Rate (per minute)	R-R Interval (sec)	Upper Limits of Normal QT Interval (sec)	
(note decreasing)	Or "Cycle Time" (note increasing)	Men (note increasing)	Women (note increasing)
150	0.4	0.25	0.28
136	0.44	0.26	0.29
125	0.48	0.28	0.3
115	0.52	0.29	0.32
107	0.56	0.3	0.33
100	0.6	0.31	0.34
93	0.64	0.32	0.35
88	0.68	0.33	0.36

78	0.72	0.35	0.38
75	0.8	0.36	0.39
71	0.84	0.37	0.4
68	0.88	0.38	0.41
65	0.92	0.38	0.42
62	0.96	0.39	0.43
60	1	0.4	0.44
57	1.04	0.41	0.45
52	1.08	0.42	0.47
50	1.2	0.44	0.48

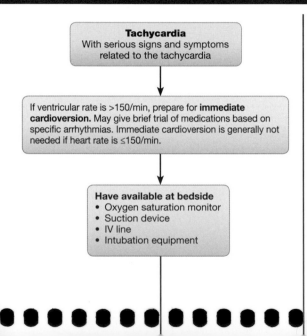

Tachycardia
With serious signs and symptoms related to the tachycardia

If ventricular rate is >150/min, prepare for **immediate cardioversion.** May give brief trial of medications based on specific arrhythmias. Immediate cardioversion is generally not needed if heart rate is ≤150/min.

Have available at bedside
- Oxygen saturation monitor
- Suction device
- IV line
- Intubation equipment

Steps for Adult Defibrillation and Cardioversion

Using Manual Defibrillators (Monophasic or Biphasic)

Assess the rhythm. If VF or pulseless VT is present, continue chest compressions without interruptions during all steps until step 8.

Defibrillation (for VF and pulseless VT)

1. Turn on defibrillator. For biphasic defibrillators, use manufacturer-specific energy if known. For monophasic defibrillators, use 360 J. If unknown, select the maximum energy available.
2. Set *lead select* switch to *paddles* (or *lead I, II,* or *III* if monitor leads are used).
3. Prepare adhesive pads (pads are preferred); if using paddles, apply appropriate conductive gel or paste. Be sure cables are attached to defibrillator.
4. Position defibrillation pads on patient's chest: one on the right anterior chest wall and one in the left axillary position. If paddles are used, apply firm pressure (about 15-25 pounds) when ready to deliver shock. If patient has an implanted pacemaker, position the pads so they are not directly over the device. Be sure that oxygen flow is not directed across the patient's chest.
5. Announce "Charging defibrillator!"
6. Press *charge* button on apex paddle or defibrillator controls.
7. When the defibrillator is fully charged, state firmly: "I am going to shock on three." Then count. "I am clear to shock!" (Chest compressions should continue until this announcement.)
8. After confirming all personnel are clear of the patient, press the *shock* button on the defibrillator or press the 2 paddle *discharge* buttons simultaneously.
9. Immediately after the shock is delivered, resume CPR beginning with compressions for 5 cycles (about 2 minutes), and then recheck rhythm. Interruption of CPR should be brief.

```
●●●●●●●●●●●●●●●●●●●  ●●●●●●●●●●●●●●●●●●●●
```

              ┌─────────────────────────────┐
              │ Premedicate whenever possible* │
              └─────────────────────────────┘
                            │
                            ▼

Synchronized cardioversion ††

Atrial fibrillation§	120-200 J, increase in stepwise fashion (per manufacturer's recommendation)
Stable monomorphic VT‖	100 J, increase in stepwise fashion (per manufacturer's recommendation)
Other SVT, atrial flutter‖	50-100 J, increase in stepwise fashion (per manufacturer's recommendation)

Notes

*Effective regimens have included a sedative (eg, diazepam, midazolam, etomidate, methohexital, propofol) with or without an analgesic agent (eg, fentanyl, morphine). Many experts recommend anesthesia if service is readily available.

†Note possible need to resynchronize after each cardioversion.

‡If delays in synchronization occur and clinical condition is critical, go immediately to unsynchronized shocks.

§These doses are for biphasic waveforms. For monophasic waveforms, initial dose is 200 J for atrial fibrillation.

‖Recommended biphasic and monophasic doses are equivalent.

Cardioversion (for tachycardia with a pulse)

Assess the rhythm. If patient has a pulse but is unstable, proceed with cardioversion.

1-4. Follow steps for defibrillation above (except for energy dose).
5. Consider sedation.
6. Engage the *synchronization* mode by pressing the *sync control* button.
7. Look for markers on R waves indicating *sync* mode is operative. If necessary, adjust monitor gain until sync markers occur with each R wave.
8. Select appropriate energy level (see Electrical Cardioversion Algorithm on left).
9. Announce "Charging defibrillator!"
10. Press *charge* button on apex paddle or defibrillator controls.
11. When the defibrillator is fully charged, state firmly: "I am going to shock on three." Then count. "I am clear to shock!"
12. After confirming all personnel are clear of the patient, press the *discharge* buttons simultaneously on paddles or the *shock* button on the unit; hold paddles in place until shock is delivered.
13. Check the monitor. If tachycardia persists, increase the energy and prepare to cardiovert again.
14. Reset the *sync* mode after each synchronized cardioversion because most defibrillators default back to unsynchronized mode. This default allows an immediate shock if the cardioversion produces VF.

Therapy	Indications/Precautions	Adult Dosage

Cardioversion
(Synchronized)

Administered via adhesive defibrillation electrode pads or handheld paddles

Place defibrillator/monitor in synchronized *(sync)* mode

Sync mode delivers energy concurrent with the QRS

Indications

- All unstable tachycardias (rate >150/min) with signs and symptoms related to tachycardia (acutely altered mental status, ischemic chest discomfort, acute heart failure, hypotension, or other signs of shock).
- A brief trial of medications is an alternative first step for specific arrhythmias.

Precautions/Contraindications

- In critical conditions, go to immediate unsynchronized shocks.
- Urgent cardioversion is generally not needed if heart rate is ≤150/min.
- Be sure oxygen is not flowing across patient's chest. Direct flow away from patient's chest and consider temporarily disconnecting bag or ventilation circuit from endotracheal tube during shock delivery.
- Reactivation of *sync* mode is required after each attempted cardioversion (defibrillator/cardioverter defaults to unsynchronized mode).
- Prepare to defibrillate immediately if cardioversion causes VF.

Technique

- Premedicate with sedatives whenever possible.
- Engage *sync* mode before each attempt.
- Look for *sync* markers on the R wave.
- Clear all personnel from the patient before each shock.
- For *regular narrow-complex tachycardias,* such as reentry SVT and atrial flutter, start with 50 J to 100 J. If initial dose fails, increase in stepwise fashion.
- For *irregular narrow-complex tachycardia* consistent with atrial fibrillation, use 200 J initial monophasic shock, or 120 to 200 J initial biphasic shock, and then increase in stepwise fashion.
- For *regular wide-complex tachycardia* consistent with monomorphic VT, start with 100 J. If initial dose fails, increase in stepwise fashion.
- *Irregular wide-complex tachycardia* consistent with unstable polymorphic VT (irregular form and rate) should be treated with high-energy *unsynchronized* dose used for VF: 360 J monophasic waveform or biphasic device-specific defibrillation dose.

(continued)

Cardioversion
(Synchronized)
(continued)

- Some defibrillators cannot deliver synchronized cardioversion unless the patient is also connected to monitor leads; in other defibrillators, ECG leads are incorporated into the defibrillation pads. Lead select switch may need to be on *lead I, II,* or *III* and not on *paddles.*

- Press *charge* button, *clear* the patient, and press both *shock* buttons simultaneously. Be prepared to perform CPR or defibrillation.

Transcutaneous Pacing

Generally external pacemakers allow adjustment of heart rate and current outputs

Indications
- Unstable bradycardia (<50/min) with signs and symptoms related to the bradycardia (hypotension, acutely altered mental status, signs of shock, ischemic chest discomfort, or acute heart failure) unresponsive to drug therapy.
- Be ready to pace in setting of AMI, as follows:
  - Markedly symptomatic sinus node dysfunction
  - Type II second-degree heart block
  - Third-degree heart block
    New left, right, or alternating BBB or bifascicular block
- Symptomatic bradycardia with ventricular escape rhythms.
- Not recommended for agonal rhythms or cardiac arrest.

Precautions
- Conscious patients may require analgesia for discomfort.
- Avoid using carotid pulse to confirm mechanical capture. Electrical stimulation causes muscular jerking that may mimic carotid pulse.

Technique
- Position pacing electrodes on chest per package instructions.
- Turn pacer on.
- Set demand rate to approximately 80/min.
- Set current (mA) output as follows for bradycardia: increase current from minimum setting until consistent capture is achieved (characterized by a widening QRS and a broad T wave after each pacer spike).

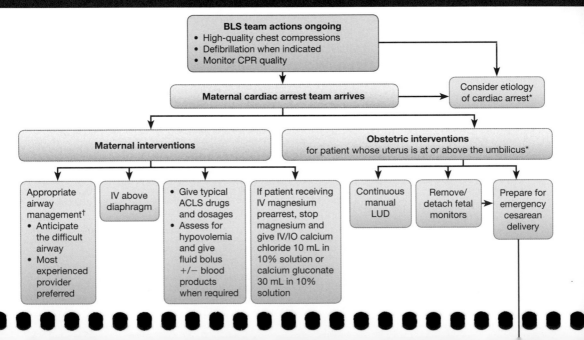

```
Neonatal team:
Prepare to
receive infant
```
→
```
If no ROSC by 4 minutes of resuscitative
efforts, consider performing immediate
emergency cesarean delivery
```

*Potential Etiology of Maternal Cardiac Arrest

A Anesthetic complications/accidents

B Bleeding

C Cardiovascular

D Drugs

E Embolic

F Fever

G General nonobstetric causes of cardiac arrest (H's and T's)

H Hypertension

†Appropriate Airway Management for Pregnancy

- 100% oxygen at ≥15 L/min and continue BLS airway strategies
- Optimally 2 attempts per technique:
  - First intubation attempt—if failed go to
  - Second intubation attempt—if failed go to
  - First supraglottic airway attempt—if failed go to
  - Second supraglottic airway attempt—if failed go to mask ventilation
  - If mask ventilation inadequate—attempt cricothyrotomy
- Avoid airway trauma
- Ventilate with 8-10 breaths/min
- Monitor capnography
- Minimize interruptions in chest compressions during advanced airway placement
- Recommend 6.0- to 7.0-mm inner diameter ETT

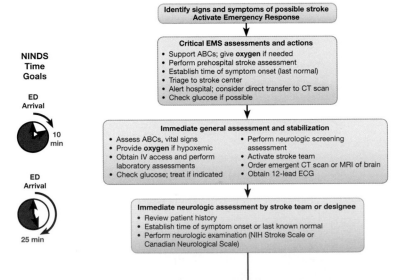

NINDS Time Goals

ED Arrival

10 min

ED Arrival

25 min

Identify signs and symptoms of possible stroke
Activate Emergency Response

Critical EMS assessments and actions
- Support ABCs; give **oxygen** if needed
- Perform prehospital stroke assessment
- Establish time of symptom onset (last normal)
- Triage to stroke center
- Alert hospital; consider direct transfer to CT scan
- Check glucose if possible

Immediate general assessment and stabilization
- Assess ABCs, vital signs
- Provide **oxygen** if hypoxemic
- Obtain IV access and perform laboratory assessments
- Check glucose; treat if indicated
- Perform neurologic screening assessment
- Activate stroke team
- Order emergent CT scan or MRI of brain
- Obtain 12-lead ECG

Immediate neurologic assessment by stroke team or designee
- Review patient history
- Establish time of symptom onset or last known normal
- Perform neurologic examination (NIH Stroke Scale or Canadian Neurological Scale)

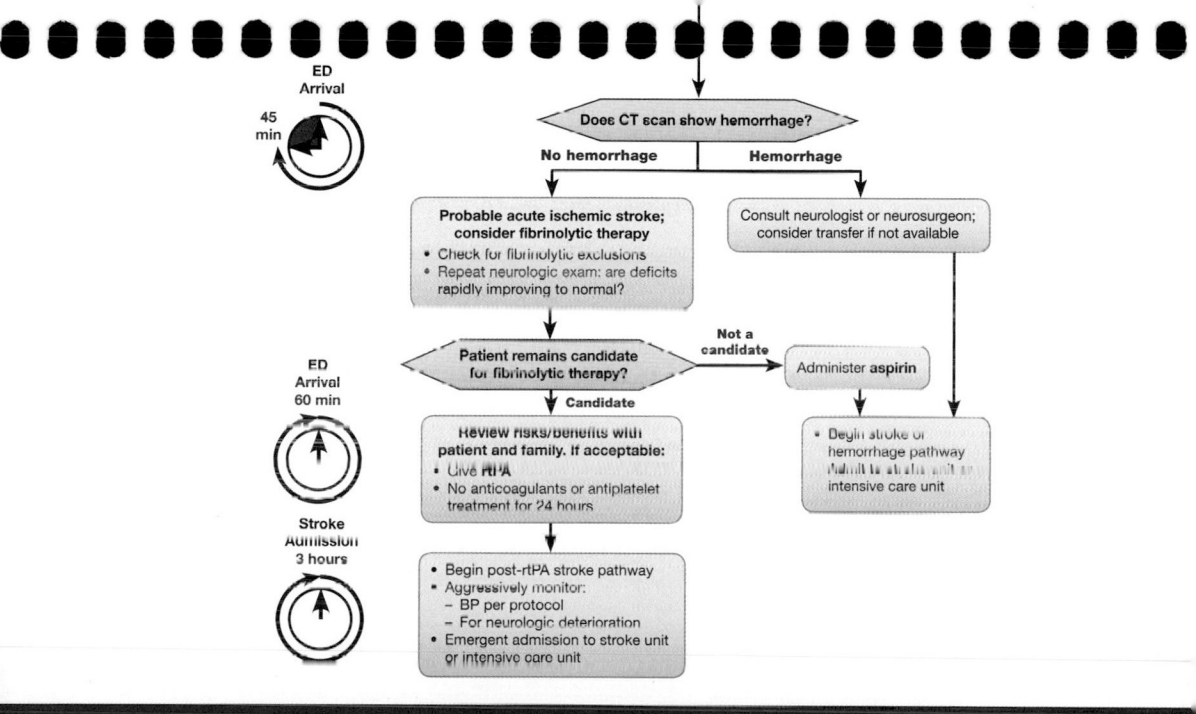

ED Arrival
45 min

Does CT scan show hemorrhage?

No hemorrhage | Hemorrhage

Probable acute ischemic stroke; consider fibrinolytic therapy
- Check for fibrinolytic exclusions
- Repeat neurologic exam: are deficits rapidly improving to normal?

Consult neurologist or neurosurgeon; consider transfer if not available

ED Arrival
60 min

Patient remains candidate for fibrinolytic therapy?

Not a candidate → Administer **aspirin**

Candidate

Review risks/benefits with patient and family. If acceptable:
- Give rtPA
- No anticoagulants or antiplatelet treatment for 24 hours

- Begin stroke or hemorrhage pathway. Admit to stroke unit or intensive care unit

Stroke Admission
3 hours

- Begin post-rtPA stroke pathway
- Aggressively monitor:
  - BP per protocol
  - For neurologic deterioration
- Emergent admission to stroke unit or intensive care unit

19

The 8 D's of Stroke Care

The 8 D's of stroke care highlight the major steps in diagnosis and treatment of stroke and key points at which delays can occur:

Detection	Rapid recognition of stroke symptoms
Dispatch	Early activation and dispatch of emergency medical services (EMS) system by calling 9-1-1
Delivery	Rapid EMS identification, management, and transport
Door	Appropriate triage to stroke center
Data	Rapid triage, evaluation, and management within the ED
Decision	Stroke expertise and therapy selection
Drug	Fibrinolytic therapy, intra-arterial strategies
Disposition	Rapid admission to stroke unit, critical care unit

Modified from Demystifying recognition and management of stroke. *Currents in Emergency Cardiac Care.* 1996;7(4):8.

Out-of-Hospital Assessment of the Patient With Acute Stroke

- Perform initial assessment
  - Assess and support airway, breathing, and circulation as needed
  - Determine level of consciousness
  - Measure vital signs frequently
- Obtain relevant history
  - Identify time of symptom onset or last seen normal
  - Determine recent illness (including history of seizures), injury, surgery, and list of medications
- Perform physical examination
  - Conduct general medical examination (including search for cardiovascular abnormalities)
  - Determine blood glucose level
  - Observe for signs of trauma
  - Conduct neurologic examination
    - Glasgow Coma Scale
    - Perform prehospital stroke screen (eg, Cincinnati Prehospital Stroke Scale, Los Angeles Prehospital Stroke Screen)
- Once possible stroke identified
  - Provide prearrival notification to receiving hospital of potential stroke patient
  - Transport rapidly to the closest available certified primary stroke center or comprehensive stroke center or, if no such centers exist, the most appropriate institution that provides emergency stroke care
  - Obtain family contact information (preferably a cell phone); bring family member or transport witness if possible

The Cincinnati Prehospital Stroke Scale

Facial Droop (have the patient show teeth or smile):
- Normal—both sides of face move equally
- Abnormal—one side of face does not move as well as the other side

Arm Drift (patient closes eyes and extends both arms straight out, with palms up, for 10 seconds):
- Normal—both arms move the same *or* both arms do not move at all (other findings, such as pronator drift, may be helpful)
- Abnormal—one arm does not move *or* one arm drifts down compared with the other

Abnormal Speech (have the patient say "you can't teach an old dog new tricks"):
- Normal—patient uses correct words with no slurring
- Abnormal—patient slurs words, uses the wrong words, or is unable to speak

Interpretation: If any 1 of these 3 signs is abnormal, the probability of a stroke is 72%.

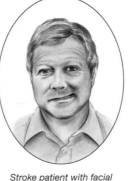

Stroke patient with facial droop (right side of face).

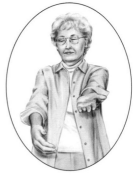

One-sided motor weakness (right arm).

Modified from Kothari RU, Pancioli A, Liu T, Brott T, Broderick J. Cincinnati Prehospital Stroke Scale: reproducibility and validity. *Ann Emerg Med.* 1999;33(4):373-378. With permission from Elsevier.

Glasgow Coma Scale*

	Score (maximum = 15)
Eye opening	
Spontaneous	4
In response to speech	3
In response to pain	2
None	1
Best verbal response	
Oriented conversation	5
Confused conversation	4
Inappropriate words	3
Incomprehensible sounds	2
None	1
Best motor response	
Obeys	6
Localizes	5
Withdraws	4
Abnormal flexion	3
Abnormal extension	2
None	1

Interpretation:

Score 14 to 15: Mild dysfunction
Score 11 to 13: Moderate to severe dysfunction
Score ≤10: Severe dysfunction

*Teasdale G, Jennett B. Assessment of coma and impaired consciousness: a practical scale. *Lancet*. 1974;2(7872):81-84.

General Management of the Acute Stroke Patient

1. **Intravenous fluids:** Avoid D_5W and excessive fluid loading. Correct hypovolemia with normal saline.

2. **Blood sugar:** Determine immediately. Bolus of 50% dextrose if hypoglycemic, insulin if serum glucose >185 mg/dL (threshold varies; check institution/system protocol).

3. **Cardiac monitoring:** During first 24 hours.

4. **Oxygen:** Pulse oximetry. Supplement for oxyhemoglobin saturation ≤94%.

5. **Acetaminophen:** If febrile (temperature >38°C).

6. **NPO:** Perform swallowing assessment.

Patients Who Could Be Treated With rtPA Within *3 Hours* From Symptom Onset*

Inclusion Criteria
- Diagnosis of ischemic stroke causing measurable neurologic deficit
- Onset of symptoms <3 hours before beginning treatment
- Age ≥18 years

Exclusion Criteria
- Head trauma or prior stroke in previous 3 months
- Symptoms suggest subarachnoid hemorrhage
- Arterial puncture at noncompressible site in previous 7 days
- History of previous intracranial hemorrhage
- Elevated blood pressure (systolic >185 mm Hg or diastolic >110 mm Hg)
- Evidence of active bleeding on examination
- Acute bleeding diathesis, including but not limited to
  - Platelet count <100 000/mm^3
  - Heparin received within 48 hours, resulting in aPTT >upper limit of normal
  - Current use of anticoagulant with INR >1.7 or PT >15 seconds
  - Current use of direct thrombin inhibitors or direct factor Xa inhibitors with elevated sensitive laboratory tests (such as aPTT, INR, platelet count, and ECT; TT; or appropriate factor Xa activity assays)
- Blood glucose concentration <50 mg/dL (2.7 mmol/L)
- CT demonstrates multilobar infarction (hypodensity >⅓ cerebral hemisphere)

Relative Exclusion Criteria

Recent experience suggests that under some circumstances—with careful consideration and weighing of risk to benefit—patients may receive fibrinolytic therapy despite 1 or more relative contraindications. Consider risk to benefit of rtPA administration carefully if any one of these relative contraindications is present:

- Only minor or rapidly improving stroke symptoms (clearing spontaneously)
- Pregnancy
- Seizure at onset with postictal residual neurologic impairments
- Major surgery or serious trauma within previous 14 days
- Recent gastrointestinal or urinary tract hemorrhage (within previous 21 days)
- Recent acute myocardial infarction (within previous 3 months)

Notes

- The checklist includes some US FDA–approved indications and contraindications for administration of rtPA for acute ischemic stroke. Recent AHA/ASA guideline revisions may differ slightly from FDA criteria. A physician with expertise in acute stroke care may modify this list.
- Onset time is either witnessed or last known normal.
- In patients without recent use of oral anticoagulants or heparin, treatment with rtPA can be initiated before availability of coagulation study results but should be discontinued if INR is > 1.7 or PT is elevated by local laboratory standards.
- In patients without history of thrombocytopenia, treatment with rtPA can be initiated before availability of platelet count but should be discontinued if platelet count is <100 000/mm^3.

Abbreviations: aPTT, activated partial thromboplastin time; CT, computed tomography; ECT, ecarin clotting time; FDA, Food and Drug Administration; INR, international normalized ratio; PT, prothrombin time; rtPA, recombinant tissue plasminogen activator; TT, thrombin time.

*Jauch EC et al. Guidelines for the early management of patients with acute ischemic stroke: a guideline for healthcare professionals from the American Heart Association/American Stroke Association. *Stroke.* 2013;44(3):870-947.

Patients Who Could Be Treated With rtPA From *3 to 4.5 Hours* From Symptom Onset[*]

Inclusion Criteria

- Diagnosis of ischemic stroke causing measurable neurologic deficit
- Onset of symptoms 3 to 4.5 hours before beginning treatment

Exclusion Criteria

- Age >80 years
- Severe stroke (NIHSS >25)
- Taking an oral anticoagulant regardless of INR
- History of both diabetes and prior ischemic stroke

Abbreviations: INR, international normalized ratio; NIHSS, National Institutes of Health Stroke Scale; rtPA, recombinant tissue plasminogen activator.

[*]del Zoppo GJ et al. Expansion of the time window for treatment of acute ischemic stroke with intravenous tissue plasminogen activator: a science advisory from the American Heart Association/American Stroke Association. *Stroke.* 2009;40(8):2945-2948.

Potential Approaches to Arterial Hypertension in Acute Ischemic Stroke Patients Who Are Potential Candidates for Acute Reperfusion Therapy*

Patient otherwise eligible for acute reperfusion therapy except that blood pressure is >185/110 mm Hg:
- Labetalol 10-20 mg IV over 1-2 minutes, may repeat × 1, or
- Nicardipine IV 5 mg per hour, titrate up by 2.5 mg per hour every 5-15 minutes, maximum 15 mg per hour; when desired blood pressure is reached, adjust to maintain proper BP limits, or
- Other agents (hydralazine, enalaprilat, etc) may be considered when appropriate

If blood pressure is not maintained at or below 185/110 mm Hg, do not administer rtPA.

Management of blood pressure during and after rtPA or other acute reperfusion therapy:
    Monitor blood pressure every 15 minutes for 2 hours from the start of rtPA therapy, then every 30 minutes for 6 hours, and then every hour for 16 hours.

If systolic blood pressure 180-230 mm Hg or diastolic blood pressure 105-120 mm Hg:
- Labetalol 10 mg IV followed by continuous IV infusion 2-8 mg per minute, or
- Nicardipine IV 5 mg per hour, titrate up to desired effect by 2.5 mg per hour every 5-15 minutes, maximum 15 mg per hour

If blood pressure not controlled or diastolic blood pressure >140 mm Hg, consider sodium nitroprusside.

Approach to Arterial Hypertension in Acute Ischemic Stroke Patients Who Are *Not* Potential Candidates for Acute Reperfusion Therapy*

Consider lowering blood pressure in patients with acute ischemic stroke if systolic blood pressure >220 mm Hg or diastolic blood pressure >120 mm Hg.

Consider blood pressure reduction as indicated for other concomitant organ system injury:
- Acute myocardial infarction
- Congestive heart failure
- Acute aortic dissection

A reasonable target is to lower blood pressure by 15% within the first 24 hours.

*Jauch EC et al. Guidelines for the early management of patients with acute ischemic stroke: a guideline for healthcare professionals from the American Heart Association/American Stroke Association. *Stroke.* 2013;44(3):870-947.

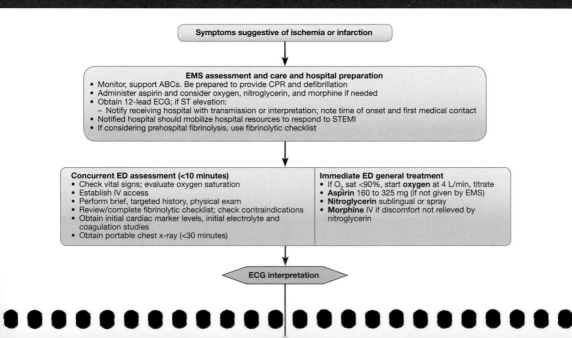

Symptoms suggestive of ischemia or infarction

EMS assessment and care and hospital preparation
- Monitor, support ABCs. Be prepared to provide CPR and defibrillation
- Administer aspirin and consider oxygen, nitroglycerin, and morphine if needed
- Obtain 12-lead ECG; if ST elevation:
  – Notify receiving hospital with transmission or interpretation; note time of onset and first medical contact
- Notified hospital should mobilize hospital resources to respond to STEMI
- If considering prehospital fibrinolysis, use fibrinolytic checklist

Concurrent ED assessment (<10 minutes)
- Check vital signs; evaluate oxygen saturation
- Establish IV access
- Perform brief, targeted history, physical exam
- Review/complete fibrinolytic checklist; check contraindications
- Obtain initial cardiac marker levels, initial electrolyte and coagulation studies
- Obtain portable chest x-ray (<30 minutes)

Immediate ED general treatment
- If O$_2$ sat <90%, start **oxygen** at 4 L/min, titrate
- **Aspirin** 160 to 325 mg (if not given by EMS)
- **Nitroglycerin** sublingual or spray
- **Morphine** IV if discomfort not relieved by nitroglycerin

ECG interpretation

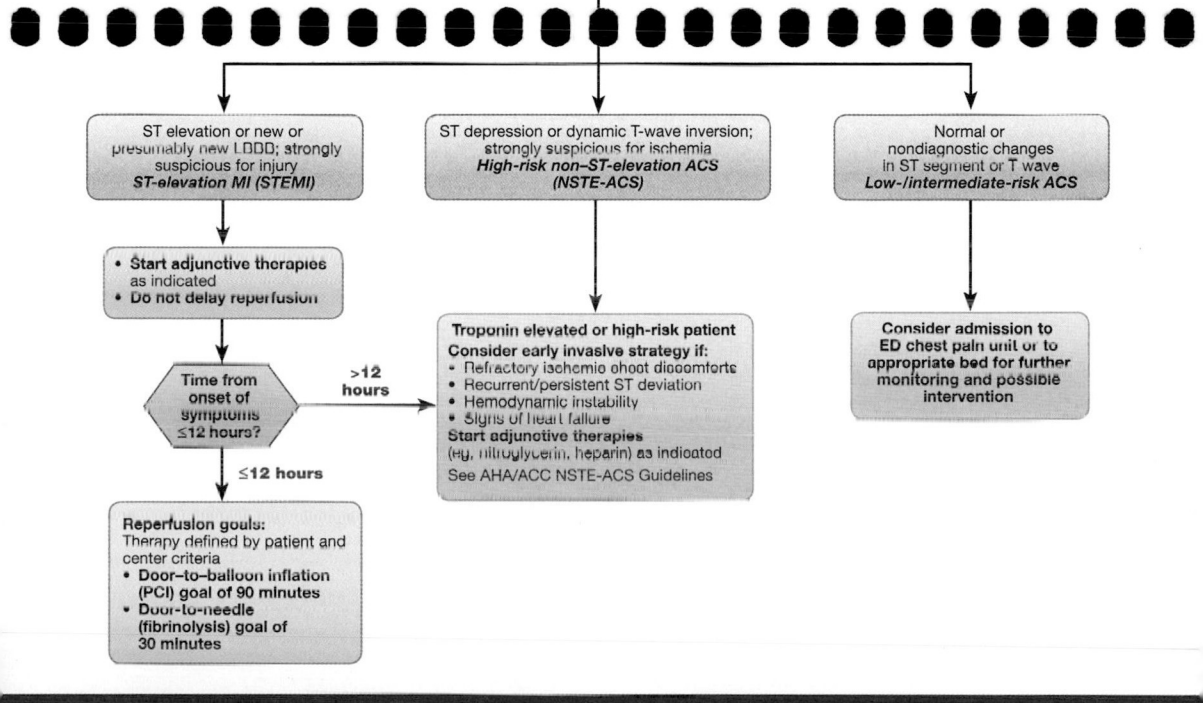

ST elevation or new or presumably new LBBB; strongly suspicious for injury
ST-elevation MI (STEMI)

ST depression or dynamic T-wave inversion; strongly suspicious for ischemia
High-risk non–ST-elevation ACS (NSTE-ACS)

Normal or nondiagnostic changes in ST segment or T wave
Low-/intermediate-risk ACS

- Start adjunctive therapies as indicated
- Do not delay reperfusion

Time from onset of symptoms ≤12 hours?

>12 hours

≤12 hours

Troponin elevated or high-risk patient
Consider early invasive strategy if:
- Refractory ischemic chest discomfort
- Recurrent/persistent ST deviation
- Hemodynamic instability
- Signs of heart failure
Start adjunctive therapies
(eg, nitroglycerin, heparin) as indicated
See AHA/ACC NSTE-ACS Guidelines

Consider admission to ED chest pain unit or to appropriate bed for further monitoring and possible intervention

Reperfusion goals:
Therapy defined by patient and center criteria
- Door–to–balloon inflation (PCI) goal of 90 minutes
- Door–to–needle (fibrinolysis) goal of 30 minutes

Likelihood That Signs and Symptoms Represent an ACS Secondary to CAD

Feature	High Likelihood *Any of the following:*	Intermediate Likelihood *Absence of high-likelihood features and presence of any of the following:*	Low Likelihood *Absence of high- or intermediate-likelihood features but may have the following:*
History	Chest or left arm pain or discomfort as chief symptom reproducing prior documented angina Known history of CAD, including MI	Chest or left arm pain or discomfort as chief symptom Age >70 years Male sex Diabetes mellitus	Probable ischemic symptoms in absence of any intermediate-likelihood characteristics Recent cocaine use
Examination	Transient MR murmur, hypotension, diaphoresis, pulmonary edema, or rales	Extracardiac vascular disease	Chest discomfort reproduced by palpation

	New or presumably new transient ST-segment deviation (≥1 mm) or T-wave inversion in multiple precordial leads	Fixed Q waves ST depression 0.5 to 1 mm or T-wave inversion >1 mm	T-wave flattening or inversion <1 mm in leads with dominant R waves Normal ECG
ECG	New or presumably new transient ST-segment deviation (≥1 mm) or T-wave inversion in multiple precordial leads	Fixed Q waves ST depression 0.5 to 1 mm or T-wave inversion >1 mm	T-wave flattening or inversion <1 mm in leads with dominant R waves Normal ECG
Cardiac markers	Elevated cardiac TnI, TnT, CK-MB, hs-TnI, or hs-TnT	Normal	Normal

Abbreviations: CAD, coronary artery disease; CK-MB, MB fraction of creatine kinase; ECG, electrocardiogram; hs, high-sensitivity; MI, myocardial infarction; MR, mitral regurgitation, TnI, troponin I; TnT, troponin T.

Anderson JL, Adams CD, Antman EM, et al. 2011 ACCF/AHA Focused Update Incorporated Into the 2007 ACC/AHA Guidelines for the Management of Patients With Unstable Angina/Non–ST-Elevation Myocardial Infarction: a report of the American College of Cardiology Foundation/American Heart Association Task Force on Practice Guidelines. *Circulation*. 2011;123(18):e426–e579. Modified from Braunwald E, Mark DB, Jones RH, et al. *Unstable Angina: Diagnosis and Management. Clinical Practice Guideline No. 10.* Rockville, MD: Agency for Health Care Policy and Research and the National Heart, Lung, and Blood Institute, Public Health Service, US Department of Health and Human Services; 1994. AHCPR publication 94-0602.

Step 1

Has patient experienced chest discomfort for greater than 15 minutes and less than 12 hours?

YES → | NO → STOP

Does ECG show STEMI or new or presumably new LBBB?

YES | NO → STOP

Step 2

Are there contraindications to fibrinolysis?
If ANY one of the following is checked YES, fibrinolysis MAY be contraindicated.

Systolic BP >180 to 200 mm Hg or diastolic BP >100 to 110 mm Hg	○ YES	○ NO
Right vs left arm systolic BP difference >15 mm Hg	○ YES	○ NO
History of structural central nervous system disease	○ YES	○ NO
Significant closed head/facial trauma within the previous 3 months	○ YES	○ NO
Stroke >3 hours or <3 months	○ YES	○ NO

Recent (within 2-4 weeks) major trauma, surgery (including laser eye surgery), GI/GU bleed	○ **YES**	○ NO
Any history of intracranial hemorrhage	○ **YES**	○ NO
Bleeding, clotting problem, or blood thinners	○ **YES**	○ NO
Pregnant female	○ **YES**	○ NO
Serious systemic disease (eg, advanced cancer, severe liver or kidney disease)	○ **YES**	○ NO

Step 3	**Is patient at high risk?** **If ANY one of the following is checked YES, consider transfer to PCI facility.**	
Heart rate ≥100/min AND systolic BP <100 mm Hg	○ **YES**	○ NO
Pulmonary edema (rales)	○ **YES**	○ NO
Signs of shock (cool, clammy)	○ **YES**	○ NO
Contraindications to fibrinolytic therapy	○ **YES**	○ NO
Required CPR	○ **YES**	○ NO

*Contraindications for fibrinolytic use in STEMI are viewed as advisory for clinical decision making and may not be all-inclusive or definitive. These contraindications are consistent with the 2004 ACC/AHA Guidelines for the Management of Patients With ST-Elevation Myocardial Infarction.

†Consider transport to primary PCI facility as destination hospital.

Evaluate for Fibrinolytic Therapy: Assess Eligibility and Risk-Benefit Ratio

Early treatment (door-to-drug time ≤30 minutes) can limit infarct size, preserve LV function, and reduce mortality.

- Maximum myocardial salvage occurs with early fibrinolytic administration, although a reduction in mortality may still be observed up to 12 hours from onset of continuous persistent symptoms.
- Normal flow achieved in 54% of patients treated with accelerated rtPA, in 33% of patients treated with streptokinase and heparin.

Most effective in the following patients:

- Early presentation
- Larger infarction
- Low risk of intracerebral hemorrhage

Benefits with age and delayed presentation:

- Patients >75 years of age have increased risk of cerebral hemorrhage but absolute benefit similar to younger patients.
- Generally not recommended if presentation 12 to 24 hours after symptom onset.

May be harmful:

- ST-segment depression (may be harmful and should not be used unless true posterior MI present)
- Patients >24 hours after onset of pain
- Number of risk factors (age [≥65 years], low body weight [<70 kg], initial hypertension [≥180/110 mm Hg]) predicts frequency of hemorrhagic stroke: no risk factors = 0.25%; 3 risk factors = 2.5%

Fibrinolytic Therapy

Contraindications for fibrinolytic use in STEMI consistent with ACC/AHA 2007 Focused Update*

Absolute Contraindications
- Any prior intracranial hemorrhage
- Known structural cerebral vascular lesion (eg, arteriovenous malformation)
- Known malignant intracranial neoplasm (primary or metastatic)
- Ischemic stroke within 3 months EXCEPT acute ischemic stroke within 3 hours
- Suspected aortic dissection
- Active bleeding or bleeding diathesis (excluding menses)
- Significant closed head trauma or facial trauma within 3 months

Relative Contraindications
- History of chronic, severe, poorly controlled hypertension
- Severe uncontrolled hypertension on presentation (SBP >180 mm Hg or DBP >110 mm Hg)†
- History of prior ischemic stroke >3 months, dementia, or known intracranial pathology not covered in contraindications
- Traumatic or prolonged (>10 minutes) CPR or major surgery (<3 weeks)
- Recent (within 2 to 4 weeks) internal bleeding
- Noncompressible vascular punctures
- For streptokinase/anistreplase: prior exposure (>5 days ago) or prior allergic reaction to these agents
- Pregnancy
- Active peptic ulcer
- Current use of anticoagulants: the higher the INR, the higher the risk of bleeding

*Viewed as advisory for clinical decision making and may not be all-inclusive or definitive.

†Could be an absolute contraindication in low-risk patients with myocardial infarction.

Alteplase, Recombinant (rtPA)

Recommended total dose is based on patient's weight.

- Accelerated infusion (1.5 hours)
  - Give 15 mg IV bolus.
  - Then 0.75 mg/kg over next 30 minutes (not to exceed 50 mg).
  - Then 0.5 mg/kg over 60 minutes (not to exceed 35 mg).
  - Maximum total dose: 100 mg.

Reteplase, Recombinant

- Give first 10 unit IV bolus over 2 minutes.
- 30 minutes later give second 10 unit IV bolus over 2 minutes. (Give NS flush before and after each bolus.)

Tenecteplase

- Bolus, weight adjusted
  - <60 kg: Give 30 mg.
  - 60-69 kg: Give 35 mg.
  - 70-79 kg: Give 40 mg.
  - 80-89 kg: Give 45 mg.
  - ≥90 kg: Give 50 mg.
- Administer single IV bolus over 5 seconds.
- Incompatible with dextrose solutions.

*See Advanced Cardiovascular Life Support Drugs section for complete details.

Immediate General Treatment
- Oxygen
- Aspirin
- Nitroglycerin
- Morphine (if unresponsive to nitrates)

Oxygen
If oxygen saturation <90% or evidence of respiratory distress: 4 L/min per nasal cannula; titrate to maintain Sao_2 ≥94%.

- **Uncomplicated MI:** Reasonable to use until stabilization. May not be helpful beyond 6 hours.

- **Complicated MI** (for overt pulmonary congestion): Administer supplementary O_2 at 4 L/min by nasal cannula; titrate as needed.

Aspirin
In either out-of-hospital or ED setting, give aspirin to all patients with ACS unless a true aspirin allergy exists (then consider clopidogrel).

Cautions and Contraindications
- Active peptic ulcer disease (use rectal suppositories).
- History of true aspirin allergy.
- Bleeding disorders, severe hepatic disease.

Recommended Dosing
- Give 160 to 325 mg non–enteric-coated orally, crushed or chewed (may use rectal suppository if cannot give by mouth).

Nitroglycerin

Indicated for patients with ischemic-type chest pain.

Cautions and Contraindications

- The use of nitrates in patients with hypotension (SBP <90 mm Hg or ≥30 mm Hg below baseline), extreme bradycardia (<50/min), or tachycardia (>100/min) in the absence of heart failure is contraindicated.
- Administer nitrates with extreme caution, if at all, to patients with inferior wall MI and suspected right ventricular involvement, because these patients require adequate RV preload. (Obtain right-sided ECG leads to assist in diagnosing RV infarct.)
- Contraindicated in patients who have recently received a phosphodiesterase inhibitor (usually given for erectile dysfunction), especially within 24 hours of sildenafil or vardenafil, or within 48 hours of tadalafil.

Recommended Dosing

- **SL:** 0.3 to 0.4 mg, repeat × 2 at 3- to 5-minute intervals, *or*
- **Spray:** 1 or 2 sprays, may repeat × 2 at 3- to 5-minute intervals, *or*
- **IV:** 12.5 to 25 mcg bolus (if no SL or spray given); then 10 mcg per minute infusion, titrated (increased at a rate of 10 mcg per minute every 3 to 5 minutes until symptom response or target arterial pressure is achieved). Ceiling dose of 200 mcg per minute commonly used.

Morphine

Indicated for patients with ischemic pain not relieved by nitroglycerin.

Cautions and Contraindications

- Do not use in patients with hypotension.
- Use cautiously in patients with suspected hypovolemia, bradycardia, or known hypersensitivity.

Recommended Dosing: STEMI

Give 2 to 4 mg IV; may give additional doses of 2 to 8 mg IV at 5- to 15-minute intervals.

Recommended Dosing: NSTE-ACS

Give 1 to 5 mg IV only if symptoms not relieved by nitrates, provided additional therapy is used to manage underlying ischemia.

Triage and Assessment of Cardiac Risk in the Emergency Department
Stratifying Patients With Possible or Probable ACS in the ED

- **Protocols must be in place to stratify** chest pain patients by risk of ACS. **The 12-lead ECG is central to ED triage of patients with ACS.** Stratify patients into one of the following subgroups (also see below):
  1. **ST-segment elevation or new LBBB:** High specificity for evolving STEMI; assess reperfusion eligibility.
  2. **ST-segment depression:** Consistent with/strongly suggestive of ischemia; defines a high-risk subset of patients with NSTE-ACS. Especially important if there are new or dynamic ECG changes. Clinical correlation is necessary to interpret completely.
  3. **Nondiagnostic or normal ECG:** Further assessment usually needed; evaluation protocols should include repeat ECG or continuous ST-segment monitoring and serial cardiac markers. Myocardial imaging or 2D echocardiogram may be useful during medical observation in selected patients. Noninvasive testing (ie, stress test/cardiac imaging) may be considered if ECG and serial markers remain normal.

- **Clinicians should carefully consider the diagnosis of ACS even in the absence of typical chest discomfort. Consider ACS in patients with**
  - Anginal equivalent symptoms, such as dyspnea (LV dysfunction), palpitations, presyncope, and syncope (ischemic ventricular arrhythmias)
  - Atypical left precordial pain or complaint of indigestion or dyspepsia
  - Atypical pain in the elderly, women, and persons with diabetes

- **Continually consider other causes of chest pain:** aortic dissection, pericarditis/myocarditis, pulmonary embolus

- **Fibrinolytic therapy:** When used for STEMI, administer within 30 minutes of hospital arrival

- **PCI:** Identify reperfusion candidates promptly and achieve balloon inflation as soon as possible with primary PCI; ideal first medical contact–to–device time system goal of ≤90 minutes if transported directly to a PCI-capable hospital and ≤120 minutes if initially seen at a non–PCI-capable hospital

Emergency Department Triage Recommendations

- **Symptoms and signs indicating need for immediate assessment and ECG within 10 minutes of presentation**
  - Chest or epigastric discomfort, nontraumatic in origin with components typical for ischemia or MI
  - Central substernal compression or crushing pain; pressure, tightness, heaviness, cramping, burning, aching sensation; unexplained indigestion, belching, epigastric pain; radiating pain in neck, jaws, shoulders, back, or one or both arms
  - Associated dyspnea, nausea or vomiting, diaphoresis
  - Palpitations, irregular pulse, or suspected arrhythmia

- **For all patients with ischemic-type chest pain**
  - Provide supplementary oxygen (until stable, for saturation <90%), IV access, and continuous ECG monitoring
  - Prompt interpretation of 12-lead ECG by physician responsible for ACS triage

- **For all patients with STEMI**
  - Initiate protocol for reperfusion therapy (fibrinolytics or PCI)
  - If fibrinolysis is planned, rule out contraindications and assess risk-benefit ratio
  - Primary PCI is the recommended method of reperfusion, including for patients considered ineligible for fibrinolytics
  - PCI (or CABG if indicated) is the preferred reperfusion treatment for patients presenting in cardiogenic shock

- **For all patients with moderate- to high-risk NSTE-ACS and STEMI**
  - Prompt aspirin (160 to 325 mg) unless given in past 24 hours
  - Clopidogrel (300 or 600 mg loading dose) or ticagrelor (180 mg loading dose); prasugrel (60 mg loading dose) may be initiated in patients proceeding to PCI after angiographic definition
  - Start adjunctive therapies (eg, nitroglycerin, heparin) as indicated. See AHA/ACC STEMI and NSTE-ACS Guidelines.

- **IV nitroglycerin for initial 24 to 48 hours only in patients with AMI and CHF, large anterior infarction, recurrent or persistent ischemia, or hypertension**

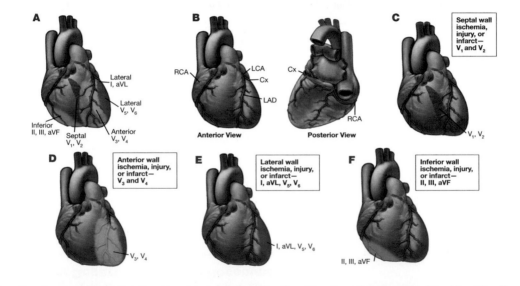

Localizing ischemia, injury, or infarct using the 12-lead ECG: relationship to coronary artery anatomy.

I lateral	aVR	V₁ septal	V₄ anterior
II inferior	aVL lateral	V₂ septal	V₅ lateral
III inferior	aVF inferior	V₃ anterior	V₆ lateral

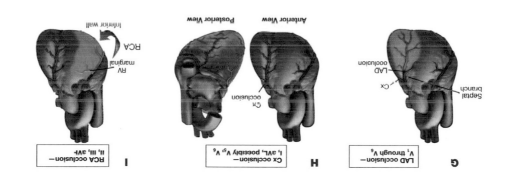

G

LAD occlusion— V₁ through V₆

Septal branch
Cx
LAD occlusion

H

Cx occlusion— I, aVL, possibly V₅, V₆

Anterior View   Posterior View

Cx occlusion

I

RCA occlusion— II, III, aVF

RV marginal
RCA
Inferior wall

How to Measure ST-Segment Deviation

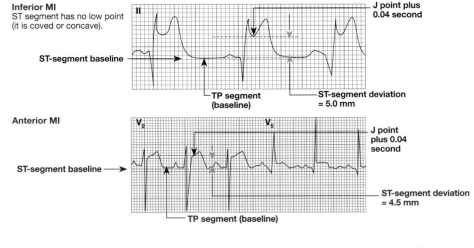

Inferior MI
ST segment has no low point (it is coved or concave).

ST-segment baseline

J point plus 0.04 second

TP segment (baseline)

ST-segment deviation = 5.0 mm

Anterior MI

V₂   V₅

ST-segment baseline

J point plus 0.04 second

ST-segment deviation = 4.5 mm

TP segment (baseline)

ECG Lead Changes Due to Injury or Infarct With Coronary Artery, Anatomical Area of Damage, and Associated Complications

Leads With ECG Changes	Injury/Infarct-Related Artery	Area of Damage	Associated Complications
V_1-V_2	LCA: LAD-septal branch	Septum, His bundle, bundle branches	Infranodal block and BBBs
V_3 V_4	LCA: LAD diagonal branch	Anterior wall LV	LV dysfunction, CHF, DDDs, complete heart block, PVCs
V_5-V_6 plus I and aVL	LCA: circumflex branch	High lateral wall LV	LV dysfunction, AV nodal block in some
II, III, aVF	RCA: posterior descending branch	Inferior wall LV, posterior wall LV	Hypotension, sensitivity to nitroglycerin and morphine sulfate
V_4R (II, III, aVF)	RCA: proximal branches	RV, inferior wall LV, posterior wall LV	Hypotension, supranodal and AV-nodal blocks, atrial fibrillation/flutter, PACs, adverse medical reactions
V_1 through V_4 (marked depression)	Either LCA-circumflex *or* RCA-posterior descending branch	Posterior wall LV	LV dysfunction

Abbreviations: AV, atrioventricular; BBB, bundle branch block; CHF, congestive heart failure; ECG, electrocardiographic; LAD, left anterior descending artery; LCA, left coronary artery; LV, left ventricle (left ventricular); PAC, premature atrial complex; PVC, premature ventricular complex; RCA, right coronary artery; RV, right ventricle.

ST-Segment Elevation or New or Presumably New LBBB: Evaluation for Reperfusion

Step 1: Assess time and risk

- Time since onset of symptoms
- Risk of STEMI (TIMI Risk Score for STEMI)
- Risk of fibrinolysis
- Time required to transport to skilled percutaneous coronary intervention (PCI) catheterization suite (first medical contact/door–to–balloon time)

Step 2: Select reperfusion (fibrinolysis or invasive) strategy

Note: If presentation ≤3 hours from symptom onset and no delay for PCI, then no preference for either strategy.

Fibrinolysis is generally preferred if:	An invasive strategy is generally preferred if:
• Early presentation (≤3 hours from symptom onset)	• Late presentation (symptom onset >3 hours ago)
• Invasive strategy is not an option (eg, lack of access to skilled PCI facility or difficult vascular access) or would be delayed • Medical contact–to–balloon or door–to–balloon time >90 min	• Skilled PCI facility available with surgical backup • Medical contact–to–balloon or door–to–balloon time <90 min
• No contraindications to fibrinolysis	• Contraindications to fibrinolysis, including increased risk of bleeding and ICH
	• High risk from STEMI (eg, presenting in shock or congestive heart failure)
	• Diagnosis of STEMI is in doubt

Evaluate for Primary PCI

Can restore vessel patency and normal flow with >90% success in experienced high-volume centers with experienced providers

Primary PCI is most effective for the following:

- In cardiogenic shock patients (<75 years old) if performed ≤18 hours from onset of shock and ≤36 hours from onset of ST-elevation infarction. However, up to 40% of shock patients require coronary artery bypass grafting (CABG) for optimal management.
- In selected patients >75 years old with STEMI and cardiogenic shock.
- In patients with indications for reperfusion but with a contraindication to fibrinolytic therapy.

Best results achieved at PCI centers with these characteristics:

- Centers with high volume (>200 PCI procedures per year; at least 36 are primary PCI)
- Experienced operator (>75 PCI procedures per year) with technical skill
- Balloon dilation <90 minutes from initial medical contact or ED presentation
- Achievement of normal flow rate (TIMI grade 3) in >90% of cases without emergency CABG, stroke, or death
  - At least 50% resolution of maximal ST-segment elevation (microvascular reperfusion)

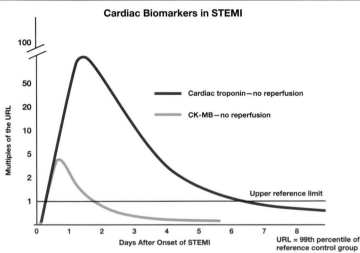

Cardiac Biomarkers in STEMI

Update: Universal Definition of AMI

- Detection of a rise and fall of cardiac biomarkers (preferably troponin) with at least 1 value above the 99th percentile of the upper reference limit (URL) and at least 1 of the following:
  - Symptoms of ischemia
  - ECG changes of ischemia: ST-T changes or new LBBB
  - Development of pathologic Q waves
  - Imaging evidence of loss of viable myocardium or new regional wall-motion abnormality

Modified from Anderson JL, et al. 2011 ACCF/AHA Focused Update Incorporated Into the ACC/AHA 2007 Guidelines for the Management of Patients With Unstable Angina/Non–ST-Elevation Myocardial Infarction: a report of the American College of Cardiology Foundation/American Heart Association Task Force on Practice Guidelines. *Circulation.* 2011;123(18):e426-e579; and Shapiro BP, Jaffe AS. Chapter 65: cardiac biomarkers. In: Murphy JG, Lloyd MA, eds. *Mayo Clinic Cardiology: Concise Textbook.* 3rd ed. Rochester, MN: Mayo Clinic Scientific Press and Informa Healthcare USA; 2007:773-779, reproduced by permission of Taylor and Francis Group, LLC, a division of Informa plc.

Cardiac Troponins

- Troponin I and troponin T are cardiac-specific structural proteins not normally detected in serum. Patients with increased troponin levels have increased thrombus burden and microvascular embolization.
- Preferred biomarker for diagnosis of MI. Increased sensitivity compared with CK-MB. Elevation above 99th percentile of mean population value is diagnostic.
- Detect minimal myocardial damage in patients with NSTE-ACS.
  - 30% of patients without ST-segment elevation who would otherwise be diagnosed with UA have small amounts of myocardial damage when troponin assays are used (eg, CK-MB negative).
  - These patients are at increased risk for major adverse cardiac events and may benefit from therapies such as GP IIb/IIIa inhibitors compared with patients who lack elevations in these cardiac-specific markers.
- Useful in risk stratification because patients with elevated serum troponin concentrations are at increased risk for subsequent nonfatal MI and sudden cardiac death.
- Can also be used to detect reinfarction.
  - Remain elevated for 7-14 days after infarct.

CK-MB

- Present in skeletal muscle and serum, less specific than troponin.
- Marker for reinfarction and noninvasive assessment of reperfusion.

TIMI Risk Score for Patients With Unstable Angina and Non–ST-Segment Elevation MI: Predictor Variables

Predictor Variable	Point Value of Variable	Definition
Age ≥65 years	1	
≥3 risk factors for CAD	1	**Risk factors:** • Family history of CAD • Hypertension • Hypercholesterolemia • Diabetes • Current smoker
Aspirin use in last 7 days	1	
Recent, severe symptoms of angina	1	≥2 anginal events in last 24 hours
Elevated cardiac markers	1	CK-MB or cardiac-specific troponin level

| ST deviation ≥0.5 mm | 1 | ST depression ≥0.5 mm is significant; transient ST elevation ≥0.5 mm for <20 minutes is treated as ST-segment depression and is high risk; ST elevation >1 mm for more than 20 minutes places these patients in the STEMI treatment category. |
| Prior coronary artery stenosis ≥50% | 1 | Risk predictor remains valid even if this information is unknown. |

Calculated TIMI Risk Score	Risk of ≥1 Primary End Point* in ≤14 Days	Risk Status
0 or 1	5%	Low
2	8%	
3	13%	Intermediate
4	20%	
5	26%	High

*Primary end points: death, new or recurrent MI, or need for urgent revascularization.

Antman EM, Cohen M, Bernink PJLM, et al. The TIMI risk score for unstable angina/non-ST elevation MI: a method for prognostication and therapeutic decision making. *JAMA.* 2000,284(7).835-842.

Global Registry of Acute Coronary Events (GRACE) Risk Model Nomogram

1. Find points for each predictive factor:

Killip Class	Points	SBP (mm Hg)	Points	Heart Rate (beats/min)	Points	Age (y)	Points	Creatinine Level (mg/dL)	Points
I	0	≤80	58	≤50	0	≤30	0	0-0.39	1
II	20	80-99	53	50-69	3	30-39	8	0.40-0.79	4
III	39	100-119	43	70-89	9	40-49	25	0.80-1.19	7
IV	59	120-139	34	90-109	15	50-59	41	1.20-1.59	10
		140-159	24	110-149	24	60-69	58	1.60-1.99	13
		160-199	10	150-199	38	70-79	75	2.00-3.99	21
		≥200	0	≥200	46	80-89	91	>4.0	28
						≥90	100		

Other Risk Factors	Points
Cardiac arrest at admission	39
ST-segment deviation	28
Elevated cardiac enzyme levels	14

2. Sum points for all predictive factors:

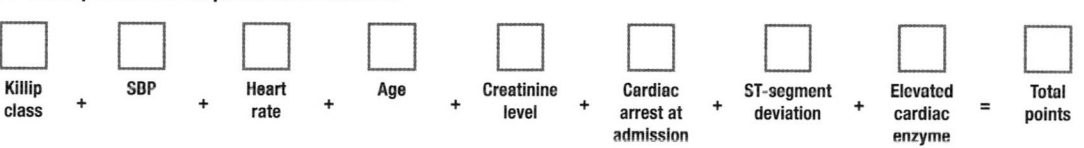

| Killip class | + | SBP | + | Heart rate | + | Age | + | Creatinine level | + | Cardiac arrest at admission | + | ST-segment deviation | + | Elevated cardiac enzyme levels | = | Total points |

3. Look up risk corresponding to total points:

Total points	<60	70	80	90	100	110	120	130	140	150	160	170	180	190	200	210	220	230	240	>250
Probability of in-hospital death (%)	≤0.2	0.3	0.4	0.6	0.8	1.1	1.6	2.1	2.9	3.9	5.4	7.3	9.8	13	18	23	29	36	44	≥52

P2Y$_{12}$ Inhibitors (also called *ADP Receptor Antagonists*)

Either clopidogrel or ticagrelor in addition to aspirin should be administered for up to 12 months to all patients with NSTE-ACS without contraindications who are treated with either an early invasive or ischemia-guided strategy.

A loading dose of a P2Y$_{12}$ inhibitor (any of the 3 below) should be given as early as possible or at the time of primary PCI to patients with STEMI or NSTE-ACS.

In patients receiving a stent during PCI for STEMI or NSTE-ACS, P2Y$_{12}$ inhibitor therapy should be given for at least 12 months.

Clopidogrel

- Aspirin and clopidogrel (300 mg loading dose for patients ≤75 years of age, 75 mg for patients >75 years of age) should be administered to patients with STEMI who receive fibrinolytic therapy.
- Aspirin should be continued indefinitely and clopidogrel (75 mg daily) should be continued for at least 14 days and up to 1 year in patients with STEMI who receive fibrinolytic therapy.
- For other indications, a loading dose of 300 to 600 mg is recommended, followed by 75 mg daily. A 600-mg loading dose results in a greater, more rapid, and more reliable platelet inhibition compared with a 300-mg loading dose.
- Clopidogrel is also recommended in patients with NSTE-ACS who are unable to take aspirin because of hypersensitivity or major gastrointestinal intolerance.
- When possible, discontinue clopidogrel at least 5 days before surgery.

Ticagrelor

- The recommended loading dose is 180 mg, followed by a maintenance dose of 90 mg twice daily.
- Compared with clopidogrel, ticagrelor has a more rapid and consistent onset of action and, because it is reversible, it has a faster recovery of platelet function. It is reasonable to choose ticagrelor over clopidogrel for $P2Y_{12}$ inhibition treatment in patients with NSTE-ACS treated with an early invasive strategy and/or coronary stenting.
- Although ticagrelor has not been studied in the absence of aspirin, its use in aspirin-intolerant patients is a reasonable alternative.
- When possible, discontinue ticagrelor at least 5 days before surgery.

Prasugrel

- The recommended loading dose is 60 mg, followed by a maintenance dose of 10 mg daily.
- Prasugrel produces more rapid and consistent platelet inhibition than clopidogrel.
- A loading dose of prasugrel is reasonable once the coronary anatomy is known in STEMI patients who did not receive a previous loading dose of clopidogrel at the time of administration of a fibrinolytic agent, but prasugrel should not be given sooner than 24 hours after administration of a fibrin-specific agent or 48 hours after administration of a non-fibrin-specific agent.
- It is reasonable to choose prasugrel over clopidogrel for treatment in patients with NSTE-ACS who undergo PCI who are not at high risk of bleeding complications
- Prasugrel is not recommended for "up-front" therapy in patients with NSTE-ACS.
- Prasugrel should not be administered to patients with a prior history of stroke or transient ischemic attack.
- When possible, discontinue prasugrel at least 5 days before surgery.

Potential Adjunctive Therapy
(Do Not Delay Reperfusion to Administer)

Anticoagulants

- **STEMI–Fibrinolytic Adjunct:** Anticoagulant therapy for a minimum of 48 hours and preferably the duration of hospitalization, up to 8 days. Regimens other than unfractionated heparin (UFH) are recommended if anticoagulant therapy is given for more than 48 hours. Recommended regimens include

  – UFH: Initial bolus 60 units/kg (maximum 4000 units) followed by intravenous infusion of 12 units/kg per hour (maximum 1000 units per hour) initially adjusted to maintain the aPTT at 50 to 70 seconds (duration of treatment 48 hours or until angiography).

  – Enoxaparin (if serum creatinine <2.5 mg/dL in men and 2 mg/dL in women): If age <75 years, an initial bolus of 30 mg IV is followed 15 minutes later by subcutaneous injections 1 mg/kg every 12 hours (maximum 100 mg for first 2 doses only). If age ≥75 years, the initial bolus is eliminated, and subcutaneous dose is reduced to 0.75 mg/kg every 12 hours (maximum 75 mg for first 2 doses only). Regardless of age, if creatinine clearance during course of treatment is estimated to be <30 mL/min (using Cockroft-Gault formula), the subcutaneous regimen is 1 mg/kg every 24 hours.

  – Patients initially treated with enoxaparin should not be switched to UFH and vice versa because of increased risk of bleeding.

  – Fondaparinux (provided serum creatinine <3 mg/dL and creatinine clearance ≥30 mL/min): Initial dose 2.5 mg IV; subsequent subcutaneous injections 2.5 mg every 24 hours. Maintenance dosing should be continued for duration of hospitalization, up to 8 days.

- **NSTE-ACS: For patients at high to intermediate risk, anticoagulant therapy should be added to antiplatelet therapy. Initial invasive strategy:**
  - UFH: Use same as above.
  - Enoxaparin: Maintenance dose: If creatinine clearance ≥30 mL/min, give 1 mg/kg subcutaneously every 12 hours. If creatinine clearance <30 mL/min, give 1 mg/kg once every 24 hours. Patients initially treated with enoxaparin should not be switched to UFH and vice versa because of increased risk of bleeding.
  - Fondaparinux: 2.5 mg subcutaneously every 24 hours. Contraindicated if creatinine clearance <30 mL/min.
  - Bivalirudin: 0.1 mg/kg bolus; maintenance 0.25 mg/kg per hour infusion.

Conveying News of a Sudden Death to Family Members

- Before talking to the family, obtain as much information as possible about the patient and the circumstances surrounding the death. Be ready to refer to the patient by name.
- Call the family if they have not been notified. Explain that their loved one has been admitted to the emergency department or critical care unit and that the situation is serious. If possible, family members should be told of the death in person, not over the telephone.
- When family members arrive, ask someone to take them to a private area. Walk in, introduce yourself, and sit down. Address the closest relative. Maintain eye contact and position yourself at the same level as family members (ie, sitting or standing).
- Enlist the aid of a social worker or a member of the clergy if possible.
- Briefly describe the circumstances leading to the death. Summarize the sequence of events. Avoid euphemisms such as "he's passed on," "she's no longer with us," or "he's left us." Instead use the words "death," "dying," or "dead."
- Allow time for family members to process the information. Make eye contact and touch. Convey your feelings with a simple phrase such as "You have my (our) sincere sympathy."
- Determine the patient's suitability for and wishes about tissue donation (use driver's license and patient records). Follow local protocols on when to discuss with family. Consent for donation should be requested by a trained individual who is not part of the care team.
- Allow as much time as necessary for questions and discussion. Review the events several times if needed.
- Allow family members the opportunity to see the patient. Prepare the family for what they will see. If equipment is still connected to the patient, tell the family. Equipment must be left in place for coroner's cases or when an autopsy is performed.
- Determine in advance what happens next and who will sign the death certificate. Physicians may impose burdens on staff and family if they fail to understand policies about death certification and disposition of the body.
- Offer to contact the patient's attending or family physician and to be available if there are further questions. Arrange for follow-up and continued support during the grieving period.

Family Presence During Resuscitation

According to surveys in the United States and the United Kingdom, most family members state that they would like to be present during the attempted resuscitation of a loved one. Parents and care providers of chronically ill patients are often knowledgeable about and comfortable with medical equipment and emergency procedures. Even family members with no medical background report that it is comforting to be at the side of a loved one and say goodbye during the final moments of life. These are those who choose to be at the bedside and who have a designated support person with them to answer questions, clarify information, and comfort the family. Family members often do not ask if they can be present, but healthcare providers should offer the opportunity whenever possible.

Relatives and friends who are present and are provided counseling during resuscitation of a loved one report fewer incidences of posttraumatic avoidance behaviors, fewer grieving symptoms, and less intrusive imagery.

When family members are present during resuscitative efforts, sensitivity is heightened among resuscitation team members. A team member who is knowledgeable about resuscitation practices should be available to answer questions, provide comfort, and help the family during the resuscitation. Even when the resuscitation outcome is not optimal, families feel comforted to know they can be present to say goodbye, give comfort to their dying loved one, and begin the grieving process.

Administration Notes

Peripheral intravenous (IV):	Resuscitation drugs administered via peripheral IV catheter should be followed by bolus of 20 mL IV fluid to move drug into central circulation. Then elevate extremity for 10 to 20 seconds.
Intraosseous (IO):	ACLS drugs that can be administered by IV route can be administered by IO route.
Endotracheal:	IV/IO administration is preferred because it provides more reliable drug delivery and pharmacologic effect. Drugs that can be administered by endotracheal route are noted in the table below. Optimal endotracheal doses have not yet been established. Medication delivered via endotracheal tube should be diluted in sterile water or NS to a volume of 5 to 10 mL. Provide several positive-pressure breaths after medication is instilled.

Drug/Therapy	Indications/Precautions	Adult Dosage
Abciximab (ReoPro)	**Indications** FDA approved for patients with NSTEMI or UA with planned PCI within 24 hours. **Precautions/Contraindications** • Binds irreversibly with platelets. Platelet function recovery requires 48 hours (regeneration). Re-administration may cause hypersensitivity reaction. • Active internal bleeding or bleeding disorder in past 30 days, history of intracranial hemorrhage or other bleeding, surgical procedure or trauma within 1 month, platelet count <150 000/mm^3, hypersensitivity and concomitant use of another GP IIb/IIIa inhibitor (also see "Acute Coronary Syndromes: Treatment Recommendations for NSTE-ACS"). • Intended for use with aspirin and heparin and has been studied in that setting only.	*Note:* **Check package insert for current indications, doses, and duration of therapy.** Optimal duration of therapy has not been established. • **PCI:** 0.25 mg/kg IV bolus (10 to 60 minutes before procedure), then 0.125 mcg/kg per minute (to maximum of 10 mcg per minute) IV infusion for 12 hours. • **Acute coronary syndrome (ACS) with planned PCI within 24 hours:** 0.25 mg/kg IV bolus, then 10 mcg per minute IV infusion for 18 to 24 hours, concluding 1 hour after PCI.

ACE (Angiotensin-Converting Enzyme) Inhibitors

Captopril

Enalapril

Lisinopril

Ramipril

Indications
- ACE inhibitors reduce mortality and improve LV dysfunction in post-AMI patients. They help prevent adverse LV remodeling, delay progression of heart failure, and decrease sudden death and recurrent MI.
- An ACE inhibitor should be administered orally within the first 24 hours after onset of AMI symptoms and continued long term if tolerated.
- Clinical heart failure without hypotension in patients not responding to digitalis or diuretics.
- Clinical signs of AMI with LV dysfunction.
- LV ejection fraction <40%.

Precautions/Contraindications for All ACE Inhibitors
- *Contraindicated* in pregnancy (may cause fetal injury or death).
- Contraindicated in angioedema.
- Hypersensitivity to ACE inhibitors.
- Reduce dose in renal failure (creatinine >2.5 mg/dL in men, >2 mg/dL in women). Avoid in bilateral renal artery stenosis.
- Serum potassium >5 mEq/l
- Do not give if patient is hypotensive (SBP <100 mm Hg or >30 mm Hg below baseline) or volume depleted.
- Generally not started in ED; after reperfusion therapy has been completed and blood pressure has stabilized, start within 24 hours.

Approach: ACE inhibitor therapy should start with low-dose oral administration (with possible IV doses for some preparations) and increase steadily to achieve a full dose within 24 to 48 hours.

An angiotensin receptor blocker (ARB) should be administered to patients intolerant of ACE inhibitors.

Captopril, AMI Dose
- Start with a single dose of 6.25 mg PO.
- Advance to 25 mg TID and then to 50 mg TID as tolerated.

Enalapril (IV = Enalaprilat)
- **PO:** Start with a single dose of 2.5 mg. Titrate to 20 mg PO BID.
- **IV:** 1.25 mg IV initial dose over 5 minutes, then 1.25 to 5 mg IV every 6 hours.
- IV form is contraindicated in STEMI (risk of hypotension).

Lisinopril, AMI Dose
- 5 mg within 24 hours of onset of symptoms, then
- 5 mg given after 24 hours, then
- 10 mg given after 48 hours, then
- 10 mg once daily

Ramipril
Start with a single dose of 2.5 mg PO. Titrate to 5 mg PO BID as tolerated.

Drug/Therapy	Indications/Precautions	Adult Dosage
Adenosine	**Indications** • First drug for most forms of stable narrow-complex SVT. Effective in terminating those due to reentry involving AV node or sinus node. • May consider for unstable narrow-complex reentry tachycardia while preparations are made for cardioversion. • Regular and monomorphic wide-complex tachycardia, thought to be or previously defined to be reentry SVT. • Does not convert atrial fibrillation, atrial flutter, or VT. • Diagnostic maneuver: stable narrow-complex SVT. **Precautions/Contraindications** • Contraindicated in poison/drug-induced tachycardia or second- or third-degree heart block. • Transient side effects include flushing, chest pain or tightness, brief periods of asystole or bradycardia, ventricular ectopy. • Less effective (larger doses may be required) in patients taking theophylline or caffeine. • Reduce initial dose to 3 mg in patients receiving dipyridamole or carbamazepine, in heart transplant patients, or if given by central venous access. • If administered for irregular, polymorphic wide-complex tachycardia/VT, may cause deterioration (including hypotension). • Transient periods of sinus bradycardia and ventricular ectopy are common after termination of SVT. • Safe and effective in pregnancy.	**IV Rapid Push** • Place patient in mild reverse Trendelenburg position before administration of drug. • Initial bolus of 6 mg given *rapidly* over 1 to 3 seconds followed by NS bolus of 20 mL; then elevate the extremity. • A second dose (12 mg) can be given in 1 to 2 minutes if needed. **Injection Technique** • Record rhythm strip during administration. • Draw up adenosine dose in one syringe and flush in another. Attach both syringes to the same or immediately adjacent IV injection ports nearest patient, with adenosine closest to patient. Clamp IV tubing above injection port. • Push IV adenosine as quickly as possible (1 to 3 seconds). • While maintaining pressure on adenosine plunger, push NS flush as rapidly as possible after adenosine. • Unclamp IV tubing.

ADP *(Adenosine Diphosphate)*
Antagonists *(Thienopyridines)*

Clopidogrel (Plavix)
Prasugrel (Effient)
Ticagrelor (Brilinta)

Indications
Adjunctive antiplatelet therapy for ACS patients.

Precautions/Contraindications
- Do not administer to patients with active pathologic bleeding (eg, peptic ulcer). Use with caution in patients with risk of bleeding.
- **Prasugrel is contraindicated in patients with a history of TIA or stroke; use with caution in patients ≥75 years old or <60 kg due to uncertain benefit and increased risk of intracranial hemorrhage and fatal bleeding.**
- Use with caution in the presence of hepatic impairment.
- **When CABG is planned, withhold ADP antagonists for 5 days (for clopidogrel and ticagrelor) or 7 days (for prasugrel) before CABG unless need for revascularization outweighs the risk of excess bleeding.**

Clopidogrel
- For STEMI or moderate to high-risk NSTE-ACS, including patients receiving fibrinolysis.
- Limited evidence in patients ≥75 years old.
- Substitute for aspirin if patient is unable to take aspirin.

Clopidogrel
- STEMI or moderate- to high-risk NSTE-ACS patients <75 years old: Administer loading dose of 300 to 600 mg orally followed by maintenance dose of 75 mg orally daily; full effects will not develop for several days.
- ED patients with suspected ACS unable to take aspirin: loading dose 300 mg.

(continued)

Drug/Therapy	Indications/Precautions	Adult Dosage
ADP Antagonists (continued)	**Prasugrel** • May be substituted for clopidogrel after angiography in patients with NSTEMI or STEMI who are not at high risk for bleeding. • Not recommended for STEMI patients managed with fibrinolysis or for NSTEMI patients before angiography. • No data to support use in ED or prehospital setting. **Ticagrelor** May be administered to patients with NSTEMI or STEMI who are treated with early invasive strategy.	**Prasugrel** • STEMI or NSTE-ACS patients <75 years old managed with PCI: Administer loading dose of 60 mg PO followed by maintenance dose of 10 mg PO daily; full effects will not develop for several days. • Consider dose reduction to 5 mg PO daily in patients weighing <60 kg. **Ticagrelor** • STEMI or NSTE-ACS patients <75 years old: Administer loading dose of 180 mg PO followed by maintenance dose 90 mg PO twice daily. • Maintenance dose of aspirin should be <100 mg/day due to drug interaction with higher doses.
Alteplase, Recombinant (Activase); **Tissue Plasminogen Activator** (rtPA) *(see Fibrinolytic Agents)*		

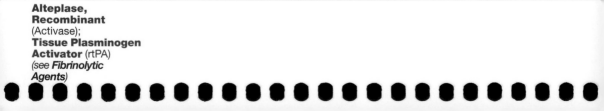

Amiodarone

Amiodarone is a complex drug with effects on sodium, potassium, and calcium channels as well as α- and β-adrenergic blocking properties. Patients must be hospitalized while the loading doses of amiodarone are administered. Amiodarone should be prescribed only by physicians who are experienced in the treatment of life-threatening arrhythmias, are thoroughly familiar with amiodarone's risks and benefits, and have access to laboratory facilities capable of adequately monitoring the effectiveness and side effects of amiodarone treatment.

Indications

Because its use is associated with toxicity, amiodarone is indicated for use in patients with life-threatening arrhythmias when administered with appropriate monitoring:

- VF/pulseless VT unresponsive to shock delivery, CPR, and a vasopressor
- Recurrent, hemodynamically unstable VT.

With expert consultation amiodarone may be used for treatment of some atrial and ventricular arrhythmias.

Caution: Multiple complex drug interactions

VF/pVT Cardiac Arrest Unresponsive to CPR, Shock, and Vasopressor

- First dose: 300 mg IV/IO push.
- Second dose (if needed): 150 mg IV/IO push.

Life-Threatening Arrhythmias

Maximum cumulative dose: 2.2 g IV over 24 hours. May be administered as follows:

- **Rapid infusion:** 150 mg IV over first 10 minutes (15 mg per minute). May repeat rapid infusion (150 mg IV) every 10 minutes as needed.
- **Slow infusion:** 360 mg IV over 6 hours (1 mg per minute).
- **Maintenance infusion:** 540 mg IV over 18 hours (0.5 mg per minute).

Precautions

- Rapid infusion may lead to hypotension.
- With multiple dosing, cumulative doses >2.2 g over 24 hours are associated with significant hypotension in clinical trials.
- Do not administer with other drugs that prolong QT interval (eg, procainamide).
- Terminal elimination is extremely long (half-life lasts up to 40 days).

Drug/Therapy	Indications/Precautions	Adult Dosage
Aspirin	**Indications** • Administer to all patients with ACS, particularly reperfusion candidates, unless hypersensitive to aspirin. • Blocks formation of thromboxane A_2, which causes platelets to aggregate and arteries to constrict. This reduces overall ACS mortality, reinfarction, and nonfatal stroke. • Any person with symptoms ("pressure," "heavy weight," "squeezing," "crushing") suggestive of ischemic pain. **Precautions/Contraindications** • Relatively contraindicated in patients with active ulcer disease or asthma. • Contraindicated in patients with known hypersensitivity to aspirin.	• Chew 160 to 325 mg tablet as soon as possible. • May use rectal suppository (300 mg) for patients who cannot take orally.

Atenolol
(see β-Blockers)

Atropine Sulfate

Can be given via endotracheal tube

Indications
- First drug for symptomatic sinus bradycardia.
- May be beneficial in presence of AV nodal block. **Not likely to be effective for type II second-degree or third-degree AV block or a block in non-nodal tissue.**
- Routine use during PEA or asystole is unlikely to have a therapeutic benefit
- Organophosphate (eg, nerve agent) poisoning: extremely large doses may be needed.

Precautions
- Use with caution in presence of myocardial ischemia and hypoxia. Increases myocardial oxygen demand.
- Unlikely to be effective for hypothermic bradycardia.
- May not be effective for infranodal (type II) AV block and new third-degree block with wide QRS complexes. (In these patients may cause paradoxical slowing. Be prepared to pace or give catecholamines.)

Bradycardia (With or Without ACS)
- 0.5 mg IV every 3 to 5 minutes as needed, not to exceed total dose of 0.04 mg/kg (total 3 mg).
- Use shorter dosing interval (3 minutes) and higher doses in severe clinical conditions.

Organophosphate Poisoning
Extremely large doses (2 to 4 mg or higher) may be needed.

Drug/Therapy	Indications/Precautions	Adult Dosage
β-Blockers **Metoprolol Tartrate** **Atenolol** **Propranolol** **Esmolol** **Labetalol** **Carvedilol**	**Indications (Apply to All β-Blockers)** • Administer to all patients with suspected myocardial infarction and unstable angina in the absence of contraindication. These are effective antianginal agents and can reduce incidence of VF. • Useful as an adjunctive agent with fibrinolytic therapy. May reduce nonfatal reinfarction and recurrent ischemia. • To convert to normal sinus rhythm or to slow ventricular response (or both) in supraventricular tachyarrhythmias (reentry SVT, atrial fibrillation, or atrial flutter). β-Blockers are second-line agents after adenosine. • To reduce myocardial ischemia and damage in AMI patients with elevated heart rate, blood pressure, or both. • Labetalol recommended for emergency antihypertensive therapy for hemorrhagic and acute ischemic stroke. **Precautions/Contraindications (Apply to All β-Blockers Unless Noted)** • Early aggressive β-blockade may be hazardous in hemodynamically unstable patients.	**Metoprolol Tartrate (AMI Regimen)** • 25 to 50 mg every 6 to 12 hours PO; then transition over next 2 to 3 days to twice-daily dosing of metoprolol tartrate or to daily metoprolol succinate; titrate to daily dose of 200 mg as tolerated. • 5 mg IV every 5 minutes as tolerated up to 3 doses; titrate to heart rate and BP. **Atenolol (AMI Regimen)** • 5 mg IV over 5 minutes. • Wait 10 minutes, then give second dose of 5 mg IV over 5 minutes. • In 10 minutes, if tolerated well, begin oral regimen with 50 mg PO; titrate to effect. **Propranolol (for SVT)** 0.5 to 1 mg over 1 minute, repeated as needed up to a total dose of 0.1 mg/kg. **Esmolol** • 0.5 mg/kg (500 mcg/kg) over 1 minute, followed by 0.05 mg/kg (50 mcg/kg) per minute infusion; maximum: 0.3 mg/kg (300 mcg/kg) per minute.

(continued)

| **β-Blockers** (continued) | • Do not give to patients with STEMI if any of the following are present:
  – Signs of heart failure.
  – Low cardiac output.
  – Increased risk for cardiogenic shock.
• Relative contraindications include PR interval >0.24 second, second- or third-degree heart block, active asthma, reactive airway disease, severe bradycardia, SBP <100 mm Hg.
• Concurrent IV administration with IV calcium channel blocking agents like verapamil or diltiazem can cause severe hypotension and bradycardia/heart block.
• Monitor cardiac and pulmonary status during administration
• Propranolol is contraindicated and other β-blockers relatively contraindicated in cocaine-induced ACS. | • If inadequate response after 5 minutes, may repeat 0.5 mg/kg (500 mcg/kg) bolus and then titrate infusion up to 0.2 mg/kg (200 mcg/kg) per minute. Higher doses unlikely to be beneficial.
• Has a short half-life (2 to 9 minutes).
Labetalol
• 10 mg IV push over 1 to 2 minutes.
• May repeat or double every 10 minutes to a maximum dose of 150 mg, or give initial dose as a bolus, then start infusion at 2 to 8 mg per minute.
Carvedilol
6.25 mg twice daily, titrate to 25 mg twice daily as tolerated. |
| **Bivalirudin** | **Indications**
This is a direct thrombin inhibitor for use in ACS.
• Useful as an anticoagulant with or without prior treatment with UFH in STEMI or NSTE-ACS patients undergoing PCI
• Preferred over UFH with GP IIb/IIIa inhibitors in patients undergoing PCI who are at high risk of bleeding.
Precautions
Reduce infusion to 1 mg/kg per hour with estimated creatinine clearance <30 mL/min. | **STEMI**
• 0.75 mg/kg IV bolus, then 1.75 mg/kg per hour infusion.
• An additional bolus of 0.3 mg/kg may be given if needed.
NSTE-ACS
• 0.10 mg/kg IV loading dose followed by 0.25 mg/kg per hour.
• Only for patients managed with an early invasive strategy.
• Continued until diagnostic angiography or PCI. |

Drug/Therapy	Indications/Precautions	Adult Dosage
Calcium Chloride 10% solution is 100 mg/mL	**Indications** • Known or suspected hyperkalemia (eg, renal failure). • Ionized hypocalcemia (eg, after multiple blood transfusions). • As an antidote for toxic effects (hypotension and arrhythmias) from calcium channel blocker overdose or β-blocker overdose. **Precautions** • Do not use routinely in cardiac arrest. • Do not mix with sodium bicarbonate.	**Typical Dose** • 500 mg to 1000 mg (5 to 10 mL of a 10% solution) IV for hyperkalemia and calcium channel blocker overdose. May be repeated as needed. • *Note:* Comparable dose of 10% calcium gluconate is 15 to 30 mL.
Captopril *(see ACE Inhibitors)*		
Clopidogrel (Plavix) *(see ADP Antagonists)*		
Digoxin-Specific Antibody Therapy Digibind (38 mg) or DigiFab (40 mg) (each vial binds about 0.5 mg digoxin) *(continued)*	**Indications** Digoxin toxicity with the following: • Life-threatening arrhythmias. • Shock or congestive heart failure. • Hyperkalemia (potassium level >5 mEq/L).	**Chronic Intoxication** 3 to 5 vials may be effective. **Acute Overdose** • IV dose varies according to amount of digoxin ingested. See "ACLS Toxicology."

Digoxin-Specific Antibody Therapy
(continued)

- Steady-state serum levels >10 to 15 ng/mL for symptomatic patients.

Precautions

Serum digoxin levels rise after digoxin antibody therapy and should not be used to guide continuing therapy.

- Average dose is 10 vials; may require up to 20 vials.
- See package insert for details.

Digoxin

0.25 mg/mL or 0.1 mg/mL supplied in 1 or 2 mL ampule (totals = 0.1 to 0.5 mg)

Indications (May Be of Limited Use)
- To slow ventricular response in atrial fibrillation or atrial flutter.
- Alternative drug for reentry SVT.

Precautions
- Toxic effects are common and are frequently associated with serious arrhythmias.
- Avoid electrical cardioversion if patient is receiving digoxin unless condition is life threatening; use lower dose (10 to 20 J).

IV Administration
- Loading doses: 0.004 to 0.006 mg/kg (4 to 6 mcg/kg) initially over 5 minutes. Second and third boluses of 0.002 to 0.003 mg/kg (2 to 3 mcg/kg) to follow at 4- to 8-hour intervals (total loading dose 8 to 12 mcg/kg divided over 8 to 16 hours).
- Check digoxin levels no sooner than 4 hours after IV dose; no sooner than 6 hours after oral dose.
- Monitor heart rate and ECG.
- Maintenance dose is affected by body mass and renal function.
- *Caution:* Amiodarone interaction. Reduce digoxin dose by 50% when used with amiodarone.

Drug/Therapy	Indications/Precautions	Adult Dosage
Diltiazem	**Indications** • To control ventricular rate in atrial fibrillation and atrial flutter. May terminate reentrant arrhythmias that require AV nodal conduction for their continuation. • Use after adenosine to treat refractory reentry SVT in patients with narrow QRS complex and adequate blood pressure. **Precautions** • Do not use calcium channel blockers for wide-QRS tachycardias of uncertain origin or for poison/drug-induced tachycardia. • Avoid calcium channel blockers in patients with Wolff-Parkinson-White syndrome plus rapid atrial fibrillation or flutter, in patients with sick sinus syndrome, or in patients with AV block without a pacemaker. • *Caution:* Blood pressure may drop from peripheral vasodilation (greater drop with verapamil than with diltiazem).	**Acute Rate Control** • 15 to 20 mg (0.25 mg/kg) IV over 2 minutes. • May give another IV dose in 15 minutes at 20 to 25 mg (0.35 mg/kg) over 2 minutes. **Maintenance Infusion** 5 to 15 mg per hour, titrated to physiologically appropriate heart rate (can dilute in D_5W or NS).

(continued)

↓

Diltiazem
(continued)

- Concurrent IV administration with IV β-blockers may produce severe hypotension. Use with extreme caution in patients receiving oral β-blockers.

Dobutamine

IV infusion

Indications

Consider for pump problems (congestive heart failure, pulmonary congestion) with SBP of 70 to 100 mm Hg and no signs of shock.

Precautions/Contraindications
- Contraindication: Suspected or known poison/drug-induced shock.
- Avoid with SBP <100 mm Hg and signs of shock.
- May cause tachyarrhythmias, fluctuations in blood pressure, headache, and nausea.
- Do not mix with sodium bicarbonate.
- Increases in heart rate of more than 10% may induce or exacerbate myocardial ischemia.

IV Administration
- Usual infusion rate is 2 to 20 mcg/kg per minute.
- Hemodynamic monitoring is recommended for optimal use.
- Elderly patients may have a significantly decreased response.

Drug/Therapy	Indications/Precautions	Adult Dosage
Dopamine IV infusion	**Indications** • Second-line drug for symptomatic bradycardia (after atropine). • Use for hypotension (SBP ≤70 to 100 mm Hg) with signs and symptoms of shock. **Precautions** • Correct hypovolemia with volume replacement before initiating dopamine. • Use with caution in cardiogenic shock with accompanying CHF. • May cause tachyarrhythmias, excessive vasoconstriction. • Do not mix with sodium bicarbonate.	**IV Administration** • Usual infusion rate is 2 to 20 mcg/kg per minute. • Titrate to patient response; taper slowly.

Enalapril
(see ACE Inhibitors)

Epinephrine

Can be given via endotracheal tube

Available in 1:10 000 and 1:1000 concentrations

Indications
- **Cardiac arrest:** VF, pulseless VT, asystole, PEA.
- **Symptomatic bradycardia:** Can be considered after atropine as an alternative infusion to dopamine.
- **Severe hypotension:** Can be used when pacing and atropine fail, when hypotension accompanies bradycardia, or with phosphodiesterase enzyme inhibitor.
- **Anaphylaxis, severe allergic reactions:** Combine with large fluid volume, corticosteroids, antihistamines.

Precautions
- Raising blood pressure and increasing heart rate may cause myocardial ischemia, angina, and increased myocardial oxygen demand.
- High doses do not improve survival or neurologic outcome and may contribute to postresuscitation myocardial dysfunction.
- Higher doses *may* be required to treat poison/drug-induced shock.

Cardiac Arrest
- **IV/IO dose:** 1 mg (10 mL of 1:10 000 solution) administered every 3 to 5 minutes during resuscitation. Follow each dose with 20 mL flush, elevate arm for 10 to 20 seconds after dose.
- **Higher dose:** Higher doses (up to 0.2 mg/kg) may be used for specific indications (β-blocker or calcium channel blocker overdose).
- **Continuous infusion.** Initial rate: 0.1 to 0.5 mcg/kg per minute (for 70-kg patient: 7 to 35 mcg per minute); titrate to response.
- **Endotracheal route:** 2 to 2.5 mg diluted in 10 mL NS.

Profound Bradycardia or Hypotension
2 to 10 mcg per minute infusion; titrate to patient response.

Drug/Therapy	Indications/Precautions	Adult Dosage
Eptifibatide	**Indications** For high-risk NSTE-ACS and patients undergoing PCI. **Actions/Precautions** Platelet function recovers within 4 to 8 hours after discontinuation. **Contraindications** Active internal bleeding or bleeding disorder in past 30 days, history of intracranial hemorrhage or other bleeding, surgical procedure or trauma within 1 month, platelet count <150 000/mm^3, hypersensitivity and concomitant use of another GP IIb/IIIa inhibitor (also see "Acute Coronary Syndromes: Treatment Recommendations for NSTE-ACS").	*Note:* **Check package insert for current indications, doses, and duration of therapy.** Optimal duration of therapy has not been established. • **PCI:** 180 mcg/kg IV bolus over 1 to 2 minutes, then begin 2 mcg/kg per minute IV infusion, then repeat bolus in 10 minutes. • Maximum dose (121-kg patient) for PCI: 22.6 mg bolus; 15 mg per hour infusion. • Infusion duration 18 to 24 hours after PCI. • Reduce rate of infusion by 50% if creatinine clearance <50 mL per minute.

Esmolol
(see β-Blockers)

Fibrinolytic Agents

Alteplase, Recombinant (Activase);
Tissue Plasminogen Activator (rtPA)

Reteplase, Recombinant (Retavase)

Tenecteplase (TNKase)

Indications

Cardiac arrest: Insufficient evidence to recommend routine use.

AMI in adults (see ACS section):
- ST elevation (threshold values: J-point elevation of 2 mm in leads V_2 and V_3* and 1 mm in all other leads) or new or presumably new LBBB.
- In context of signs and symptoms of AMI.
- Time from onset of symptoms <12 hours.
- See "Acute Coronary Syndromes: Fibrinolytic Checklist for STEMI" and Fibrinolytic Therapy under "ST Segment Elevation Therapies: Fibrinolytic Strategy" for guidance on use of fibrinolytics in patients with STEMI.

Acute ischemic stroke (see Stroke section). (Alteplase is the only fibrinolytic agent approved for acute ischemic stroke.)
- Sudden onset of focal neurologic deficits or alterations in consciousness (eg, facial droop, arm drift, abnormal speech).

*Threshold value of 2.5 mm in men <40 years; 1.5 mm in all women.

For all 4 agents, insert 2 peripheral IV lines; use 1 line exclusively for fibrinolytic administration.

Alteplase, Recombinant (rtPA)
50- and 100-mg vials reconstituted with sterile water to 1 mg/mL.

Recommended total dose is based on patient's weight.

STEMI:
- Accelerated infusion (1.5 hours)
  - Give 15 mg IV bolus.
  - Then 0.75 mg/kg over next 30 minutes (not to exceed 50 mg).
  - Then 0.5 mg/kg over 60 minutes (not to exceed 35 mg).
  - Maximum total dose: 100 mg.

Acute ischemic stroke:
- Give 0.9 mg/kg (maximum 90 mg) IV, infused over 60 minutes.
- Give 10% of total dose as an initial IV bolus over 1 minute.
- Give remaining 90% of total dose IV over next 60 minutes.

(continued)

Drug/Therapy	Indications/Precautions	Adult Dosage

Fibrinolytic Agents *(continued)*	• See "Use of IV rtPA for Acute Ischemic Stroke: Inclusion and Exclusion Characteristics" for guidance on which patients can be treated with rtPA based on time of symptom onset.
	
	Precautions and Possible Exclusion Criteria for AMI in Adults/Acute Ischemic Stroke
	• For AMI in adults, see "Acute Coronary Syndromes: Fibrinolytic Checklist for STEMI" and Fibrinolytic Therapy under "ST-Segment Elevation Therapies: Fibrinolytic Strategy" for indications, precautions, and contraindications.
	• For acute ischemic stroke, see "Use of IV rtPA for Acute Ischemic Stroke: Inclusion and Exclusion Characteristics" for indications, precautions, and contraindications.
		Reteplase, Recombinant
		10-unit vials reconstituted with sterile water to 1 unit/mL.
		• Give first 10-unit IV bolus over 2 minutes.
		• 30 minutes later give second 10-unit IV bolus over 2 minutes. (Give NS flush before and after each bolus.)
		
		Tenecteplase
		50-mg vial reconstituted with sterile water
		• Bolus, weight adjusted
		  — <60 kg: Give 30 mg.
		  — 60-69 kg: Give 35 mg.
		  — 70-79 kg: Give 40 mg.
		  — 80-89 kg: Give 45 mg.
		  — ≥90 kg: Give 50 mg.
		• Administer single IV bolus over 5 seconds.
		• Incompatible with dextrose solutions.

Flumazenil

Indications
Reverse respiratory depression and sedative effects from pure benzodiazepine overdose.

Precautions
- Effects may not outlast effect of benzodiazepines.
- Monitor for recurrent respiratory depression.
- Do not use in suspected tricyclic overdose.
- Do not use in seizure-prone patients, chronic benzodiazepine users, or alcoholics.
- Do not use in unknown drug overdose or mixed drug overdose with drugs known to cause seizures (tricyclic antidepressants, cocaine, amphetamines, etc).

First Dose
0.2 mg IV over 15 seconds.

Second Dose
0.3 mg IV over 30 seconds. If no adequate response, give third dose.

Third Dose
0.5 mg IV given over 30 seconds. If no adequate response, repeat once every minute until adequate response or a total of 3 mg is given.

Drug/Therapy	Indications/Precautions	Adult Dosage
Fondaparinux (Arixtra)	**Indications** • For use in ACS. • To inhibit thrombin generation by factor Xa inhibition. • May be used for anticoagulation in patients with history of heparin-induced thrombocytopenia. **Precautions/Contraindications** • Hemorrhage may complicate therapy. • Contraindicated in patients with creatinine clearance <30 mL per minute; use with caution in patients with creatinine clearance 30 to 50 mL per minute. **Increased risk of catheter thrombosis in patients undergoing PCI; coadministration of unfractionated heparin required.**	**STEMI Protocol** Initial dose 2.5 mg IV bolus followed by 2.5 mg subcutaneously every 24 hours for up to 8 days. **NSTE-ACS Protocol** 2.5 mg subcutaneously every 24 hours.

Furosemide

Indications
- For adjuvant therapy of acute pulmonary edema in patients with SBP >90 to 100 mm Hg (without signs and symptoms of shock).
- Hypertensive emergencies.

Precautions
Dehydration, hypovolemia, hypotension, hypokalemia, or other electrolyte imbalance may occur.

IV Administration
- 0.5 to 1 mg/kg given over 1 to 2 minutes.
- If no response, double dose to 2 mg/kg, given slowly over 1 to 2 minutes.
- For new-onset pulmonary edema with hypovolemia: <0.5 mg/kg.

Glucagon

Powdered in 1-mg vials

Reconstitute with provided solution

Indications
Adjuvant treatment of toxic effects of calcium channel blocker or β-blocker.

Precautions
May cause vomiting, hyperglycemia.

IV Infusion
3 to 10 mg IV slowly over 3 to 5 minutes, followed by infusion of 3 to 5 mg per hour.

Drug/Therapy	Indications/Precautions	Adult Dosage
Glycoprotein IIb/IIIa Inhibitors		
Abciximab (ReoPro)		
Eptifibatide (Integrilin)		
Tirofiban (Aggrastat)		
(See individual drug listings for indications, precautions, and contraindications.)		

Heparin, Unfractionated (UFH)

Concentrations range from 1000 to 40 000 units/mL

Indications
- Adjuvant therapy in AMI.
- Begin heparin with fibrin-specific lytics (eg, alteplase, reteplase, tenecteplase).

Precautions/Contraindications
- Same contraindications as for fibrinolytic therapy: active bleeding; recent intracranial, intraspinal, or eye surgery; severe hypertension; bleeding disorders; gastrointestinal bleeding.
- Doses and laboratory targets appropriate when used with fibrinolytic therapy.
- Do not use if platelet count is or falls below <100 000 or with history of heparin-induced thrombocytopenia. For these patients, consider direct antithrombins.

UFH IV Infusion—STEMI
- Initial bolus 60 units/kg (maximum bolus: 4000 units).
- Continue 12 units/kg per hour, round to the nearest 50 units (maximum initial rate: 1000 units per hour).
- Adjust to maintain aPTT 1.5 to 2 times the control values for 48 hours or until angiography
- Check initial aPTT at 3 hours, then every 6 hours until stable, then daily.
- Follow institutional heparin protocol.
- Platelet count daily.

UFH IV Infusion—NSTE-ACS
- Initial bolus 60 units/kg. Maximum: 4000 units.
- 12 units/kg per hour. Maximum initial rate: 1000 units per hour.
- Follow institutional protocol (see Heparin in ACS section).

Drug/Therapy	Indications/Precautions	Adult Dosage
Heparin, Low Molecular Weight (LMWH)	**Indications** For use in ACS, specifically patients with NSTE-ACS. These drugs inhibit thrombin generation by factor Xa inhibition and also inhibit thrombin indirectly by formation of a complex with antithrombin III. These drugs are **not** neutralized by heparin-binding proteins. **Precautions** • Hemorrhage may complicate any therapy with LMWH. Contraindicated in presence of hypersensitivity to heparin or pork products or history of sensitivity to drug. Use LMWH with extreme caution in patients with type II heparin-induced thrombocytopenia. • Adjust dose for renal insufficiency. • Contraindicated if platelet count <100 000. For these patients, consider direct antithrombins. **Heparin Reversal** For ICH or life-threatening bleed: Administer protamine; refer to package insert.	**STEMI Protocol** • Enoxaparin — Age <75 years, normal creatinine clearance: Initial bolus 30 mg IV with second bolus 15 minutes later of 1 mg/kg subcutaneously; repeat every 12 hours (maximum 100 mg/dose for first 2 doses). — Age ≥75 years: Eliminate initial IV bolus; give 0.75 mg/kg subcutaneously every 12 hours (maximum 75 mg/dose for first 2 doses). — If creatinine clearance <30 mL per minute, give 1 mg/kg subcutaneously every 24 hours. **NSTE-ACS Protocol** Enoxaparin: Loading dose 30 mg IV bolus. Maintenance dose 1 mg/kg subcutaneously every 12 hours. If creatinine clearance <30 mL per minute, give every 24 hours.

Ibutilide

Intervention of choice is DC cardioversion

Indications

Treatment of supraventricular arrhythmias, including atrial fibrillation and atrial flutter when duration ≤48 hours. Short duration of action. Effective for the conversion of atrial fibrillation or flutter of relatively brief duration.

Precautions/Contraindications

Contraindication: Do not give to patients with QT_c >440 milliseconds. Ventricular arrhythmias develop in approximately 2% to 5% of patients (polymorphic VT, including torsades de pointes). *Monitor ECG continuously for arrhythmias during administration and for 4 to 6 hours after administration with defibrillator nearby.* Patients with significantly impaired LV function are at highest risk for arrhythmias.

Dose for Adults ≥60 kg

1 mg (10 mL) administered IV (diluted or undiluted) over 10 minutes. A second dose may be administered at the same rate 10 minutes later.

Dose for Adults <60 kg

0.01 mg/kg initial IV dose administered over 10 minutes.

Drug/Therapy	Indications/Precautions	Adult Dosage
Isoproterenol IV infusion	**Indications** • *Use cautiously as temporizing measure if external pacer is not available* for treatment of symptomatic bradycardia. • Refractory torsades de pointes unresponsive to magnesium sulfate. • *Temporary* control of bradycardia in heart transplant patients (denervated heart unresponsive to atropine). • Poisoning from β-blockers. **Precautions** • Do not use for treatment of cardiac arrest. • Increases myocardial oxygen requirements, which may increase myocardial ischemia. • Do not give with epinephrine; can cause VF/pVT. • Do not give to patients with poison/drug-induced shock (except for β-blocker poisoning). • May use higher doses for β-blocker poisoning.	**IV Administration** • Infuse at 2 to 10 mcg per minute. • Titrate to adequate heart rate. • In torsades de pointes, titrate to increase heart rate until VT is suppressed.
Labetalol *(see β-Blockers)*		

Lidocaine

Can be given via endotracheal tube

Indications
- Alternative to amiodarone in cardiac arrest from VF/pVT.
- Stable monomorphic VT with preserved ventricular function.
- Stable polymorphic VT with normal baseline QT interval and preserved LV function when ischemia is treated and electrolyte balance is corrected.
- Can be used for stable polymorphic VT with baseline QT interval prolongation if torsades suspected.

Precautions/Contraindications
- Contraindication: *Prophylactic* use in AMI is contraindicated.
- Reduce maintenance dose (not loading dose) in presence of impaired liver function or LV dysfunction.
- Discontinue infusion immediately if signs of toxicity develop

Cardiac Arrest From VF/pVT
- Initial dose: 1 to 1.5 mg/kg IV/IO.
- For refractory VF, may give additional 0.5 to 0.75 mg/kg IV push and repeat in 5 to 10 minutes; maximum 3 doses or total of 3 mg/kg.

Perfusing Arrhythmia
For stable VT, wide-complex tachycardia of uncertain type, significant ectopy.
- Doses ranging from 0.5 to 0.75 mg/kg and up to 1 to 1.5 mg/kg may be used.
- Repeat 0.5 to 0.75 mg/kg every 5 to 10 minutes; maximum total dose: 3 mg/kg.

Maintenance Infusion
1 to 4 mg per minute (30 to 50 mcg/kg per minute).

Lisinopril
(see ACE Inhibitors)

Drug/Therapy	Indications/Precautions	Adult Dosage
Magnesium Sulfate	**Indications** • Recommended for use in cardiac arrest only if torsades de pointes or suspected hypomagnesemia is present. • Life-threatening ventricular arrhythmias due to digitalis toxicity. • Routine administration in hospitalized patients with AMI is not recommended. **Precautions** • Occasional fall in blood pressure with rapid administration. • Use with caution if renal failure is present.	**Cardiac Arrest** **(Due to Hypomagnesemia or Torsades de Pointes)** 1 to 2 g (2 to 4 mL of a 50% solution diluted in 10 mL [eg, D$_5$W, normal saline] given IV/IO). **Torsades de Pointes With a Pulse or AMI With Hypomagnesemia** • Loading dose of 1 to 2 g mixed in 50 to 100 mL of diluent (eg, D$_5$W, normal saline) over 5 to 60 minutes IV. • Follow with 0.5 to 1 g per hour IV (titrate to control torsades).
Mannitol Strengths: 5%, 10%, 15%, 20%, and 25%	**Indications** Increased intracranial pressure in management of neurologic emergencies. **Precautions** • Monitor fluid status and serum osmolality (not to exceed 310 mOsm/kg). • Caution in renal failure because fluid overload may result.	**IV Administration** • Administer 0.5 to 1 g/kg over 5 to 10 minutes through in-line filter. • Additional doses of 0.25 to 2 g/kg can be given every 4 to 6 hours as needed. • Use with support of oxygenation and ventilation.

Metoprolol Tartrate
(see β-Blockers)

Milrinone

Indications

Myocardial dysfunction and increased systemic or pulmonary vascular resistance, including
- Congestive heart failure in postoperative cardiovascular surgical patients
- Shock with high systemic vascular resistance.

Precautions

May produce nausea, vomiting, hypotension, particularly in volume-depleted patients. Drug may accumulate in renal failure and in patients with low cardiac output; reduce dose in renal failure.

Loading Dose

50 mcg/kg over 10 minutes IV loading dose.

IV Infusion
- 0.375 to 0.75 mcg/kg per minute.
- Hemodynamic monitoring required.
- Reduce dose in renal impairment.

Drug/Therapy	Indications/Precautions	Adult Dosage
Morphine Sulfate	**Indications** • Chest pain with ACS unresponsive to nitrates. • Acute cardiogenic pulmonary edema (if blood pressure is adequate). **Precautions** • Administer slowly and titrate to effect. • May cause respiratory depression. • Causes hypotension in volume-depleted patients. • Use with caution in RV infarction. • May reverse with naloxone (0.04 to 2 mg IV).	**IV Administration** • STEMI: Give 2 to 4 mg IV. May give additional doses of 2 to 8 mg IV at 5- to 15-minute intervals. Analgesic of choice. • NSTE-ACS: Give 1 to 5 mg IV only if symptoms not relieved by nitrates or if symptoms recur. Use with caution.

Naloxone Hydrochloride

Can be given via endotracheal tube

Indications

Respiratory and neurologic depression due to opiate intoxication unresponsive to oxygen and support of ventilation.

Precautions

- May cause severe opiate withdrawal, including hypertensive crisis and pulmonary edema when given in large doses (titration of small doses recommended)
- Half-life shorter than narcotics; repeat dosing may be needed.
- Monitor for recurrent respiratory depression.
- Rare anaphylactic reactions have been reported.
- Assist ventilation before naloxone administration; avoid sympathetic stimulation.
- Avoid in meperidine-induced seizures.

Administration

- Typical IV dose 0.04 to 0.4 mg; titrate until ventilation adequate.
- Use higher doses for complete narcotic reversal.
- Can administer up to 6 to 10 mg over short period (<10 minutes).
- If total reversal is not required (eg, respiratory depression from sedation), smaller doses of 0.04 mg repeated every 2 to 3 minutes may be used.
- For chronic opioid addicted patients, use smaller dose and titrate slowly.

Opioid-Associated Life-Threatening Emergencies

- **IM or IV:** 0.04 to 0.4 mg, repeated every 2 to 3 minutes if necessary.
- **Intranasal:** 2 mg, repeated every 3 to 5 minutes if necessary.

Advanced Cardiovascular Life Support Drugs

Drug/Therapy	Indications/Precautions	Adult Dosage
Nicardipine (Cardene) Calcium channel blocker	**Indications** • Hypertensive emergencies. • Decrease blood pressure to ≤185/110 mm Hg before administration of fibrinolytic therapy. **Precautions/Contraindications** • Avoid rapid decrease in blood pressure. • Reflex tachycardia or increased angina may occur in patients with extensive coronary disease. • Avoid use in patients with severe aortic stenosis. • Do not mix with sodium bicarbonate or Ringer's lactate solution.	**Acute Hypertension Emergencies** • Initial infusion rate 5 mg per hour; may increase by 2.5 mg per hour every 5 to 15 minutes to maximum of 15 mg per hour. • Decrease infusion rate to 3 mg per hour once desired blood pressure reached.
Nitroglycerin Available in IV form, sublingual tablets, and aerosol spray	**Indications** • Initial antianginal for suspected ischemic pain. • For initial 24 to 48 hours in patients with *AMI and CHF*, large anterior wall infarction, persistent or recurrent ischemia, or hypertension.	**IV Administration** • **IV bolus:** 12.5 to 25 mcg (if no SL or spray given).

(continued)

Nitroglycerin
(continued)

- Continued use (beyond 48 hours) for patients with recurrent angina or persistent pulmonary congestion (nitrate-free interval recommended).
- Hypertensive urgency with ACS.

Contraindications
- Hypotension (SBP <90 mm Hg or ≥30 mm Hg below baseline).
- Severe bradycardia (<50 per minute) or tachycardia (>100 per minute).
- RV infarction.
- Use of phosphodiesterase inhibitors for erectile dysfunction (eg, sildenafil and vardenafil within 24 hours; tadalafil within 48 hours).

Precautions
- Generally, with evidence of AMI and normotension, do not reduce SBP to <110 mm Hg. If patient is hypertensive, do not decrease mean arterial pressure (MAP) by >25% (from initial MAP).
- Do not mix with other drugs.
- Patient should sit or lie down when receiving this medication.
- Do not shake aerosol spray because this affects metered dose.

- **Infusion:** Begin at 10 mcg per minute. Titrate to effect; increase by 10 mcg per minute every 3 to 5 minutes until desired effect. Ceiling dose of 200 mcg per minute commonly used.
  — Route of choice for emergencies.

Sublingual Route
- 1 tablet (0.3 to 0.4 mg), repeated for total of 3 doses at 5-minute intervals
- 1 to 2 sprays at 5-minute intervals (provides 0.4 mg per dose). Maximum 3 sprays within 15 minutes.
- *Note:* Patients should be instructed to contact EMS if pain is unrelieved or increasing after 1 tablet or sublingual spray.

Drug/Therapy	Indications/Precautions	Adult Dosage
Nitroprusside (Sodium Nitroprusside)	**Indications** • Hypertensive crisis. • To reduce afterload in heart failure and acute pulmonary edema. • To reduce afterload in acute mitral or aortic valve regurgitation. **Precautions** • May cause hypotension and cyanide toxicity. • May reverse hypoxic pulmonary vasoconstriction in patients with pulmonary disease, exacerbating intrapulmonary shunting, resulting in hypoxemia. • Other side effects include headaches, nausea, vomiting, and abdominal cramps. • Contraindicated in patients who have recently taken phosphodiesterase inhibitors for erectile dysfunction (eg, sildenafil).	**IV Administration** • Begin at 0.1 mcg/kg per minute and titrate upward every 3 to 5 minutes to desired effect (usually up to 5 mcg/kg per minute, but higher doses up to 10 mcg/kg may be needed). • Use with an infusion pump; use hemodynamic monitoring for optimal safety. • Action occurs within 1 to 2 minutes. • Light sensitive; cover drug reservoir and tubing with opaque material.

Norepinephrine

Indications

- Severe cardiogenic shock and hemodynamically significant hypotension (SBP <70 mm Hg) with low total peripheral resistance.
- Agent of last resort for management of ischemic heart disease and shock.

Precautions

- Increases myocardial oxygen requirements; raises blood pressure and heart rate.
- May induce arrhythmias. Use with caution in patients with acute ischemia; monitor cardiac output.
- Extravasation causes tissue necrosis.
- If extravasation occurs, administer phentolamine 5 to 10 mg in 10 to 15 mL saline solution; infiltrate into area.
- Relatively contraindicated in patients with hypovolemia.

IV Administration (Only Route)

- Initial rate: 0.1 to 0.5 mcg/kg per minute (for 70-kg patient: 7 to 35 mcg per minute); titrate to response.
- Do not administer in same IV line as alkaline solutions.
- Poison/drug-induced hypotension may require higher doses to achieve adequate perfusion.

Drug/Therapy	Indications/Precautions	Adult Dosage

Oxygen

Delivered from portable tanks or installed, wall-mounted sources through delivery devices

Indications
- Any suspected cardiopulmonary emergency.
- Complaints of shortness of breath and suspected ischemic pain.
- For ACS: May administer to all patients until stable. Continue if pulmonary congestion, ongoing ischemia, or oxygen saturation <94%.
- For patients with suspected stroke and hypoxemia, arterial oxygen desaturation (oxyhemoglobin saturation <94%), or unknown oxyhemoglobin saturation. May consider administration to patients who are not hypoxemic.
- After ROSC following resuscitation: Use the minimum inspired oxygen concentration to achieve oxyhemoglobin saturation ≥94%. If equipment available, to avoid hyperoxia, wean inspired oxygen when oxyhemoglobin saturation is 100% but maintain ≥94%.

Device	Flow Rate	O_2 (%)
Nasal cannula	1-6 L per minute	21-44
Venturi mask	4-12 L per minute	24-50
Partial rebreathing mask	6-10 L per minute	35-60
Nonrebreathing oxygen mask with reservoir	6-15 L per minute	60-100
Bag-mask with nonrebreathing "tail"	15 L per minute	95-100

Note: Pulse oximetry provides a useful method of titrating oxygen administration to maintain physiologic oxygen saturation (see Precautions).

(continued)

Oxygen
(continued)

Precautions
- Observe closely when using with pulmonary patients known to be dependent on hypoxic respiratory drive (very rare).
- Pulse oximetry may be inaccurate in low cardiac output states, with vasoconstriction, or with exposure to carbon monoxide.

Prasugrel (Effient)
(see ADP Antagonists)

Drug/Therapy	Indications/Precautions	Adult Dosage

Procainamide	**Indications**
	• Useful for treatment of a wide variety of arrhythmias, including stable monomorphic VT with normal QT interval and preserved LV function.
	• May use for treatment of reentry SVT uncontrolled by adenosine and vagal maneuvers if blood pressure stable.
	• Stable wide-complex tachycardia of unknown origin.
	• Atrial fibrillation with rapid rate in Wolff-Parkinson-White syndrome.
	
	Precautions
	• If cardiac or renal dysfunction is present, reduce maximum total dose to 12 mg/kg and maintenance infusion to 1 to 2 mg per minute.
	• Proarrhythmic, especially in setting of AMI, hypokalemia, or hypomagnesemia.
	• May induce hypotension in patients with impaired LV function.
	• Use with caution with other drugs that prolong QT interval (eg, amiodarone). Expert consultation advised.
		Recurrent VF/pVT
		• 20 mg per minute IV infusion (maximum total dose: 17 mg/kg).
		• In urgent situations, up to 50 mg per minute may be administered to total dose of 17 mg/kg.
		
		Other Indications
		• 20 mg per minute IV infusion until one of the following occurs:
		  — Arrhythmia suppression.
		  — Hypotension.
		  — QRS widens by >50%.
		  — Total dose of 17 mg/kg is given.
		• Use in cardiac arrest limited by need for slow infusion and uncertain efficacy.
		
		Maintenance Infusion
		1 to 4 mg per minute (dilute in D_5W or NS). Reduce dose in presence of renal or hepatic insufficiency.

Propranolol
(see β-Blockers)

Ramipril
(see ACE Inhibitors)

**Reteplase,
Recombinant**
(Retavase)
(see Fibrinolytic Agents)

Drug/Therapy	Indications/Precautions	Adult Dosage
Sodium Bicarbonate	**Indications** • Known preexisting hyperkalemia. • Known preexisting bicarbonate-responsive acidosis; eg, diabetic ketoacidosis or overdose of tricyclic antidepressant, aspirin, cocaine, or diphenhydramine. • Prolonged resuscitation with effective ventilation; on return of spontaneous circulation after long arrest interval. • Not useful or effective in hypercarbic acidosis (eg, cardiac arrest and CPR without intubation). **Precautions** • Adequate ventilation and CPR, not bicarbonate, are the major "buffer agents" in cardiac arrest. • Not recommended for routine use in cardiac arrest patients.	**IV Administration** • 1 mEq/kg IV bolus. • If rapidly available, use arterial blood gas analysis to guide bicarbonate therapy (calculated base deficits or bicarbonate concentration). During cardiac arrest, ABG results are not reliable indicators of acidosis.

Sotalol

Seek expert consultation

Indications

Treatment of supraventricular arrhythmias and ventricular arrhythmias in patients without structural heart disease.

Precautions/Contraindications

- Should be avoided in patients with poor perfusion because of significant negative inotropic effects.
- Adverse effects include bradycardia, hypotension, and arrhythmias (torsades de pointes).
- Use with caution with other drugs that prolong QT interval (eg, procainamide, amiodarone).
- May become toxic in patients with renal impairment; contraindicated if creatinine clearance <40 mL per minute.

IV Administration

- 1 to 1.5 mg/kg.
- Check hospital protocol for infusion rate. Package insert recommends slow infusion, but literature supports more rapid infusion of 1.5 mg/kg over 5 minutes or less.

Tenecteplase
(TNKase)

(see Fibrinolytic Agents)

Drug/Therapy	Indications/Precautions	Adult Dosage

Thienopyridines
(see ADP Antagonists)

Thrombolytic Agents
(see Fibrinolytic Agents)

Ticagrelor (Brilinta)
(see ADP Antagonists)

Tirofiban (Aggrastat)

Indications
For high-risk NSTE-ACS and patients undergoing PCI.

Actions/Precautions
Platelet function recovers within 4 to 8 hours after discontinuation.

Contraindications
Active internal bleeding or bleeding disorder in past 30 days, history of intracranial hemorrhage or other bleeding, surgical procedure or trauma within 1 month, platelet count <150 000/mm^3, hypersensitivity and concomitant use of another GP IIb/IIIa inhibitor (also see "Acute Coronary Syndromes: Treatment Recommendations for NSTE-ACS").

Note: **Check package insert for current indications, doses, and duration of therapy.** Optimal duration of therapy has not been established.

- **PCI:** 25 mcg/kg administered over 3 minutes; then 0.15 mcg/kg per minute IV infusion (for 18 to 24 hours after PCI).
- Reduce rate of infusion by 50% if creatinine clearance <60 mL per minute.

Drug/Therapy	Indications/Precautions	Adult Dosage
Vasopressin	**Indications** May be useful for hemodynamic support in vasodilatory shock (eg, septic shock). **Precautions/Contraindications** • Potent peripheral vasoconstrictor. Increased peripheral vascular resistance may provoke cardiac ischemia and angina. • Not recommended for responsive patients with coronary artery disease.	**IV Administration** **Vasodilatory shock:** Continuous infusion of 0.02 to 0.04 units per minute.

Verapamil

Indications
- Alternative drug (after adenosine) to terminate reentry SVT with narrow QRS complex and adequate blood pressure and *preserved LV function*.
- May control ventricular response in patients with atrial fibrillation, flutter, or multifocal atrial tachycardia.

Precautions
- Give *only* to patients with narrow-complex reentry SVT or known supraventricular arrhythmias.
- Do not use for wide-QRS tachycardias of uncertain origin, and avoid use for Wolff-Parkinson-White syndrome and atrial fibrillation, sick sinus syndrome, or second- or third-degree AV block without pacemaker.
- May decrease myocardial contractility, and can produce peripheral vasodilation and hypotension. IV calcium may restore blood pressure in toxic cases.
- Concurrent IV administration with IV β-blockers may produce severe hypotension. Use with extreme caution in patients receiving oral β-blockers.

IV Administration
- **First dose:** 2.5 to 5 mg IV bolus over 2 minutes (over 3 minutes in older patients).
- **Second dose:** 5 to 10 mg, if needed, every 15 to 30 minutes. Maximum total dose: 20 mg.
- **Alternative:** 5 mg bolus every 15 minutes to total dose of 30 mg.

Useful Calculations and Formulas

Calculation	Formula	Comments
Anion gap (serum concentration in mEq/L)	$[Na^+] - ([Cl^-] + [HCO_3^-])$	Normal range: 10 to 15 mEq/L. A gap >15 suggests a high anion gap metabolic acidosis.
Osmolal gap	$Osmolality_{measured} - Osmolality_{calculated}$ Normal = <10	Osmolal gap normally <10 suggests a high anion gap metabolic acidosis. If osmolal gap is >10, suspect unknown osmotically active substances.
Calculated osmolality (in mOsm/L)	$(2 \times [Na^+]) + ([Glucose] \div 18) + ([BUN] \div 2.8)$	Simplified to give *effective* osmolality. Normal = 272 to 300 mOsm/L

Determination of *predicted* pH	$(40 - P_{CO_2}) \times 0.008 = \pm\Delta$ in pH from 7.4	For every 1 mm Hg uncompensated change in P_{CO_2} from 40, pH will change by 0.008.
		Measured pH less than predicted pH: metabolic acidosis is present.
		Measured pH greater than predicted pH: metabolic alkalosis is present.

Emergency Treatments and Treatment Sequence for Hyperkalemia

Therapy	Dose	Effect Mechanism	Onset of Effect	Duration of Effect
Calcium	• Calcium chloride (10%): 5 to 10 mL IV • Calcium gluconate (10%): 15 to 30 mL IV	Antagonism of toxic effects of hyperkalemia at cell membrane	1 to 3 min	30 to 60 min
Sodium bicarbonate	• Begin with 50 mEq IV • May repeat in 15 minutes	Redistribution: intracellular shift	5 to 10 min	1 to 2 h
Insulin plus glucose (use 2 units insulin per 5 g glucose)	10 units regular insulin IV plus 25 g dextrose (50 mL D_{50})	Redistribution: intracellular shift	30 min	4 to 6 h

Nebulized albuterol	• 10 to 20 mg over 15 min • May repeat	Redistribution: intracellular shift	15 min	15 to 90 min
Diuresis with furosemide	40 to 80 mg IV bolus	Removal from body	At start of diuresis	Until end of diuresis
Cation-exchange resin (Kayexalate)	15 to 50 g PO or PR plus sorbitol	Removal from body	1 to 2 h	4 to 6 h
Peritoneal or hemodialysis	Per institutional protocol	Removal from body	At start of dialysis	Until end of dialysis

Common Toxidromes*

Whenever possible, contact a medical toxicologist or poison center (eg, in USA: 1-800-222-1222) for advice when treating suspected severe poisoning.

Cardiac Signs		
Tachycardia and/or Hypertension • Amphetamines • Anticholinergic drugs • Antihistamines • Cocaine • Theophylline/caffeine • Withdrawal states	**Bradycardia and/or Hypotension** • β-Blockers • Calcium channel blockers • Clonidine • Digoxin and related glycosides • Organophosphates and carbamates	**Cardiac Conduction Delays (Wide QRS)** • Cocaine • Cyclic antidepressants • Local anesthetics • Propoxyphene • Vaughan-Williams Class Ia and Ic agents (eg, quinidine, flecainide)
CNS/Metabolic Signs		
Seizures • Cyclic antidepressants • Isoniazid • Selective and nonselective norepinephrine reuptake inhibitors (eg, bupropion) • Withdrawal states	**CNS and/or Respiratory Depression** • Antidepressants (several classes) • Benzodiazepines • Carbon monoxide • Ethanol • Methanol • Opioids • Oral hypoglycemics	**Metabolic Acidosis** • Cyanide • Ethylene glycol • Iron • Metformin • Methanol • Salicylates

*Differential diagnosis lists are partial.

Rapid Dosing Guide for Antidotes Used in Emergency Cardiovascular Care for Treatment of Toxic Ingestions

Whenever possible, consult a medical toxicologist or call poison center (eg, in USA: 1-800-222-1222) for advice before administering antidotes.

Antidote	Common Indications: Toxicity due to	Adult Dose*	Pediatric Dose* *Do not exceed adult dose*	Notes
Atropine	• β-Blockers • Calcium channel blockers • Clonidine • Digoxin	0.5-1 mg IV every 2-3 minutes	0.02 mg/kg IV (minimum dose 0.1 mg) every 2-3 minutes	Use for hemodynamically significant bradycardia. Higher doses often required for organo-phosphate or carbamate poisoning.
Calcium	• β-Blockers • Calcium channel blockers	• Calcium chloride (10%): 1-2 g (10-20 mL) IV • Calcium gluconate (10%): 3-6 g (30-60 mL) IV • Follow initial dose with same dose by continuous hourly infusion	• Calcium chloride (10%). 20 mg/kg (0.2 mL/kg) IV • Calcium gluconate (10%): 60 mg/kg (0.6 mL/kg) IV • Follow initial dose with same dose by continuous hourly infusion	Use for hypotension. Avoid calcium chloride when possible if using peripheral IV, particularly in children. Higher doses may be required for calcium channel blocker overdose (use caution and monitor serum calcium).

*These doses are often different from doses used in other emergency cardiovascular care situations. The ideal dose has not been determined for many indications; the doses above may not be ideal. Most antidotes may be repeated as needed to achieve and maintain the desired clinical effect. Unless otherwise noted, IV doses may also be given via the IO route. Contact medical toxicologist, call poison center (eg, in USA: 1-800-222-1222), or refer to written treatment guidance for specific dosing advice.

(continued)

Rapid Dosing Guide for Antidotes Used in Emergency Cardiovascular Care for Treatment of Toxic Ingestions *(continued)*

Antidote	Common Indications: Toxicity due to	Adult Dose*	Pediatric Dose* *Do not exceed adult dose*	Notes
Digoxin Immune Fab	• Digoxin and related glycosides	• **If amount of digoxin ingested is known:** Give 1 vial IV for every 0.5 mg digoxin ingested. • **If amount of digoxin ingested is unknown or if chronic intoxication with a known digoxin level:** Dose (vials, administered IV) = $\frac{\text{(serum digoxin concentration [ng/mL]} \times \text{weight [kg])}}{100}$ • **Unknown dose and level, cardiovascular collapse:** 10-20 vials IV		
Flumazenil	• Benzodiazepines	0.2 mg IV every 15 seconds, up to 3 mg total dose	0.01 mg/kg IV every 15 seconds, up to 0.05 mg/kg total dose	Do not use for unknown overdose, suspected TCA overdose, or patients who are benzodiazepine dependent due to risk of precipitating seizures.
Glucagon	• β-Blockers • Calcium channel blockers	3-10 mg IV bolus, followed by 3-5 mg per hour IV infusion	0.05-0.15 mg/kg IV bolus, followed by 0.05-0.10 mg/kg per hour IV infusion	Bolus often causes vomiting.

Hydroxo-cobalamin	• Cyanide	5 g IV	70 mg/kg IV	Dilute in 100 mL normal saline; infuse over 15 minutes. Toxicologist or other specialist may follow with sodium thiosulfate (separate IV).
Lipid Emulsion	• Local anesthetics • Possibly other toxicants if failing standard resuscitation	1.5 mL/kg lean body mass of 20% emulsion of long-chain triglycerides IV bolus over 1 minute followed by infusion of 0.25 mL/kg per minute for 30 to 60 minutes. The bolus can be repeated once or twice as needed for persistent cardiovascular collapse; suggested maximum total dose is 10 mL/kg over first hour.		
Insulin	• β-Blockers • Calcium channel blockers	1 unit/kg IV bolus, then 0.5-1 units/kg per hour IV infusion, titrated to blood pressure		Give dextrose 0.5 g/kg with insulin. Start dextrose infusion 0.5 g/kg per hour and check blood sugar frequently. Replace potassium to maintain serum potassium 2.5-2.8 mEq/L.

*These doses are often different from doses used in other emergency cardiovascular care situations. The ideal dose has not been determined for many indications; the doses above may not be ideal. Most antidotes may be repeated as needed to achieve and maintain the desired clinical effect. Unless otherwise noted, IV doses may also be given via the IO route. Contact medical toxicologist, call poison center (eg, in USA: 1-800-222-1222), or refer to written treatment guidance for specific dosing advice.

(continued)

Rapid Dosing Guide for Antidotes Used in Emergency Cardiovascular Care for Treatment of Toxic Ingestions (continued)

Antidote	Common Indications: Toxicity due to	Adult Dose*	Pediatric Dose* *Do not exceed adult dose*	Notes
Naloxone	• Opioids	• IM or IV: 0.04-0.4 mg, repeated every 2-3 minutes if necessary • Intranasal: 2 mg, repeated every 3-5 minutes if necessary	0.1 mg/kg IV (up to 2 mg per dose). Repeat every 2-3 minutes. For partial reversal of respiratory depression (eg, procedural sedation), 0.001-0.005 mg/kg (1-5 mcg/kg) IV. Titrate to effect.	Use only for respiratory depression or loss of airway reflexes. May also be given by IO, nebulized, or endotracheal routes.
Sodium Bicarbonate	• Cyclic antidepressants	1 mEq/kg IV (1 mL/kg of 8.4% solution); consider infusion following initial dose		Repeat as needed until QRS narrows. Avoid sodium >155 mEq/L or pH >7.55. Dilute before administration in small children.

Sodium Nitrite	• Cyanide	300 mg IV over 3-5 minutes (10 mL of 3% solution)	10 mg/kg (0.33 mL/kg of 10% solution) IV over 3-5 minutes	Hydroxocobalamin preferred to sodium nitrite, if available. May give inhaled amyl nitrite as temporizing measure while establishing vascular access. Follow with sodium thiosulfate administration. Reduced dose required for children with anemia.
Sodium Thiosulfate	• Cyanide	12.5 g (50 mL of 25% solution) IV over 10 minutes	400 mg/kg (1.65 mL/kg of 25% solution) IV over 10 minutes	Use separate IV from hydroxocobalamin. Consider expert consultation.

These doses are often different from doses used in other emergency cardiovascular care situations. The ideal dose has not been determined for many indications; the doses above may not be ideal. Most antidotes may be repeated as needed to achieve and maintain the desired clinical effect. Unless otherwise noted, IV doses may also be given via the IO route. Contact medical toxicologist, call poison center (eg, in USA: 1-800-222-1222), or refer to written treatment guidance for specific dosing advice.

Pre-event Equipment Checklist for Endotracheal Intubation

☐	Universal precautions (gloves, mask, eye protection)
☐	Cardiac monitor, pulse oximeter, and blood pressure monitoring device
☐	Continuous waveform capnography device or, if not available, exhaled CO_2 detector (qualitative) or esophageal detector device (aspiration technique)
☐	Intravenous and intraosseous infusion equipment
☐	Oxygen supply, bag mask (appropriate size)
☐	Oral/tracheal suction equipment (appropriate size); confirm that it is working
☐	Oral and nasopharyngeal airways (appropriate size)
☐	Endotracheal tubes with stylets (all sizes) and sizes 0.5 mm (i.d.) above and below anticipated size for patient
☐	Laryngoscope (curved and straight blades) and/or video laryngoscope; backup laryngoscope available
☐	10-mL syringes to test inflate endotracheal tube balloon
☐	Adhesive/cloth tape or commercial endotracheal tube holder to secure tube
☐	Towels, sheets, or pad to align airway by placing under head or torso
☐	Rescue equipment as needed for difficult airway management or anticipated complications (eg, supraglottic airway, transtracheal ventilation, and/or cricothyrotomy equipment)

Pre-event preparation	1. Obtain brief medical history and perform focused physical examination. 2. Prepare equipment, monitors, personnel, medications. 3. If neck injury not suspected: place in sniffing position. If neck injury suspected: stabilize cervical spine.
Preoxygenate	4. Preoxygenate with FiO_2 of 100% by mask (nonrebreather preferred). If ventilatory assistance is necessary, ventilate gently.
Premedicate	5. Premedicate as appropriate; wait briefly to allow adequate drug effect after administration.
Pharmacologic sedation/anesthesia/ neuromuscular blockade and protection/positioning	6. Administer sedation/anesthesia by IV push. 7. Give neuromuscular blocking agent by IV push. 8. Apply cricoid pressure. 9. Assess for apnea, jaw relaxation, and absence of movement (patient sufficiently relaxed to proceed with intubation).
Placement of endotracheal tube	10. Perform endotracheal intubation. If during intubation oxygen saturation is inadequate, stop laryngoscopy and start ventilation with bag-mask. Monitor pulse oximetry and ensure adequate oxygen saturation. Reattempt intubation. Once intubated, inflate cuff to minimal occlusive volume. Be prepared to place rescue airway if intubation attempts are unsuccessful.
Placement confirmation	11. Confirm placement of endotracheal tube by • direct visualization of ET passing through vocal cords • chest rise/fall with each ventilation (bilateral) • 5-point auscultation: anterior chest L and R, midaxillary line L and R, and over the epigastrium (no breath sounds over epigastrium); look for tube condensation • using end-tidal CO_2 measured by quantitative continuous waveform capnography; If waveform capnography not available, use qualitative exhaled CO_2 detector or esophageal detector device (aspiration technique) • monitoring O_2 saturation (indirect evidence of adequate oxygenation)
Postintubation management	12. Prevent dislodgement: • Secure ET with adhesive/cloth tape or commercial ET holder • Continue cervical spine immobilization • Continue sedation; add paralytics if necessary • Check cuff inflation pressure

Pharmacologic Agents Used for Rapid Sequence Intubation

Drug	IV/IO Push*	Onset	Duration	Side Effects	Comments
Premedication Agents					
Atropine	0.01-0.02 mg/kg (minimum: 0.1 mg; maximum single dose: 0.5 mg)	1-2 min	2-4 hours	Paradoxical bradycardia can occur with doses <0.1 mg Tachycardia, agitation	Antisialogogue Inhibits bradycardic response to hypoxia, laryngoscopy, and succinylcholine May cause pupil dilation
Glycopyrrolate	0.005-0.01 mg/kg (maximum: 0.2 mg)	1-2 min	4-6 hours	Tachycardia	Antisialogogue Inhibits bradycardic response to hypoxia, laryngoscopy, and succinylcholine
Lidocaine	1-2 mg/kg (maximum: 100 mg)	1-2 min	10-20 min	Myocardial and CNS depression Seizures with high doses	May decrease ICP during RSI May decrease pain on propofol injection

Sedative/Anesthetic Agents					
Etomidate	0.2-0.4 mg/kg Caution: Limit to 1 dose	<1 min	5-10 min	Myoclonic activity Inhibition of cortisol synthesis for up to 12 hours	Ultrashort acting No analgesic properties Decreases cerebral metabolic rate and ICP Generally maintains hemodynamic stability
Fentanyl citrate	2-5 mcg/kg	1-3 min	30-60 min	Chest wall rigidity possible with high-dose rapid infusions	Minimum histamine release May lower blood pressure (especially with higher doses or in conjunction with midazolam)
Ketamine	1-2 mg/kg	30-60 sec	10-20 min	Hypertension, tachycardia Increased secretions and laryngospasm Emergence reactions and hallucinations	Dissociative anesthetic agent Limited respiratory depression Bronchodilator May cause myocardial depression in catecholamine-depleted patients Use with caution in patients with potential or increased ICP

Abbreviations: BP, blood pressure; CNS, central nervous system; ICP, intracranial pressure; IO, intraosseous; IV, intravascular.

*Doses provided are guidelines only. Actual dosing may vary depending on patient's clinical status.

(continued)

Pharmacologic Agents Used for Rapid Sequence Intubation *(continued)*

Drug	IV/IO Push*	Onset	Duration	Side Effects	Comments
Sedative/Anesthetic Agents *(continued)*					
Midazolam	0.1-0.3 mg/kg (maximum single dose: 10 mg)	2-5 min	15-30 min	Hypotension	Hypotension exacerbated in combination with narcotics and barbiturates No analgesic properties Excellent amnesia
Propofol	1-2 mg/kg	<1 min	5-10 min	Hypotension, especially in patients with inadequate intravascular volume Pain on infusion	No analgesic properties Very short duration of action Less airway reactivity than barbiturates Decreases cerebral metabolic rate and ICP Lidocaine may decrease infusion pain Not recommended in patients with egg/soy allergy

Drug	IV/IO Dose*	Time to Paralysis	Duration of Paralysis	Side Effects	Comments
Neuromuscular Blocking Agents					
Succinylcholine	1-1.5 mg/kg	45-60 sec	5-10 min	Muscle fasciculations May cause rhabdomyolysis; rise in intracranial, intraocular, intragastric pressure; life-threatening hyperkalemia	Depolarizing muscle relaxant Rapid onset, short duration of action Avoid in burns, crush injuries after 48 hours, muscular dystrophy and other neuromuscular diseases, hyperkalemia, or family history of malignant hyperthermia Use with caution in renal failure; monitor serum potassium Do *not* use to maintain paralysis
Vecuronium	0.1-0.2 mg/kg	1-3 min	45-90 min	Minimal cardiovascular side effects	Nondepolarizing agent The higher the dose, the quicker the onset of action and the longer the duration
Cisatracurium	0.4 mg/kg	2-3 min	90-120 min	Minimal cardiovascular side effects	Nondepolarizing agent Degrades spontaneously, independent of organ elimination
Rocuronium	0.6-1.2 mg/kg	60-90 sec	45-120 min	Minimal cardiovascular side effects	Nondepolarizing agent Rapid onset of action

Abbreviations: ICP, intracranial pressure; IO, intraosseous; IV, intravascular.

*Doses provided are guidelines only. Actual dosing may vary depending on patient's clinical status.

Capnography to Confirm Endotracheal Tube Placement

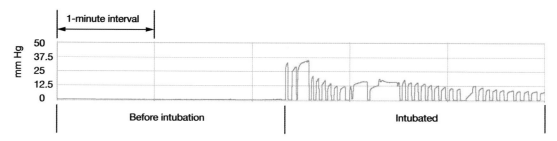

This capnography tracing displays the partial pressure of exhaled carbon dioxide ($PETCO_2$) in mm Hg on the vertical axis over time when intubation is performed. Once the patient is intubated, exhaled carbon dioxide is detected, confirming tracheal tube placement. The $PETCO_2$ varies during the respiratory cycle, with highest values at end-expiration.

Capnography to Monitor Effectiveness of Resuscitation Efforts

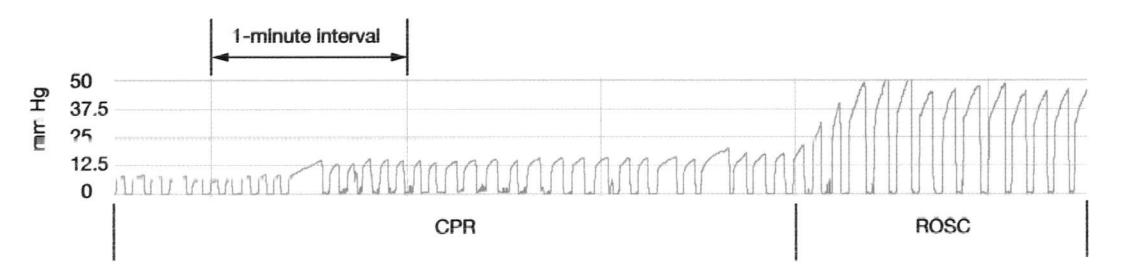

This second capnography tracing displays the P_{ETCO_2} in mm Hg on the vertical axis over time. This patient is intubated and receiving CPR. Note that the ventilation rate is approximately 8-10 breaths per minute. Chest compressions are given continuously at a rate of slightly faster than 100/min but are not visible with this tracing. The initial P_{ETCO_2} is less than 12.5 mm Hg during the first minute, indicating very low blood flow. The P_{ETCO_2} increases to between 12.5 and 25 mm Hg during the second and third minutes, consistent with the increase in blood flow with ongoing resuscitation. Return of spontaneous circulation (ROSC) occurs during the fourth minute. ROSC is recognized by the abrupt increase in the P_{ETCO_2} (visible just after the fourth vertical line) to over 40 mm Hg, which is consistent with a substantial improvement in blood flow.

Newborn Resuscitation

Ideally, newborn resuscitation takes place in the delivery room or the neonatal intensive care unit, with trained personnel and appropriate equipment readily available. This form of resuscitation is taught in the **Neonatal Resuscitation Program (NRP)** offered by the American Academy of Pediatrics and the AHA. These pages provide information about initial assessment of the newborn and initial stabilization priorities. *Ensuring adequate ventilation of the baby's lungs is the most important and effective action in neonatal resuscitation.*

Initial Assessment and Stabilization

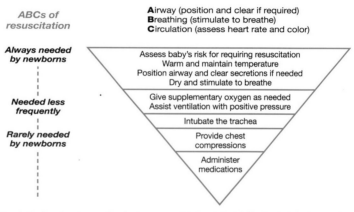

ABCs of resuscitation

Airway (position and clear if required)
Breathing (stimulate to breathe)
Circulation (assess heart rate and color)

Always needed by newborns

Assess baby's risk for requiring resuscitation
Warm and maintain temperature
Position airway and clear secretions if needed
Dry and stimulate to breathe

Needed less frequently

Give supplementary oxygen as needed
Assist ventilation with positive pressure

Intubate the trachea

Rarely needed by newborns

Provide chest compressions

Administer medications

A majority of newborns respond to simple measures. The inverted pyramid reflects relative frequencies of resuscitative efforts for a newborn who does not have meconium-stained amniotic fluid.

Targeted Preductal SpO$_2$ After Birth

1 min	60%-65%	4 min	75%-80%
2 min	65%-70%	5 min	80%-85%
3 min	70%-75%	10 min	85%-95%

The ranges shown are approximations of the interquartile values reported by Mariani et al and are adjusted to provide easily remembered targets.

Mariani G, Dik PB, Ezquer A, et al. Pre-ductal and post-ductal O$_2$ saturation in healthy term neonates after birth. *J Pediatr.* 2007;150(4):418-421.

Apgar Score

Sign	0	1	2
Color	Blue or pale	Acrocyanotic	Completely pink
Heart rate	Absent	<100/min	>100/min
Reflex irritability	No response	Grimace	Cry or active withdrawal
Muscle tone	Limp	Some flexion	Active motion
Respiration	Absent	Weak cry; hypoventilation	Good, crying

From Kattwinkel J, ed. Lesson 1: Overview and Principles of Resuscitation. *Textbook of Neonatal Resuscitation.* 6th ed. Elk Grove Village, IL: American Academy of Pediatrics and American Heart Association; 2011:35.

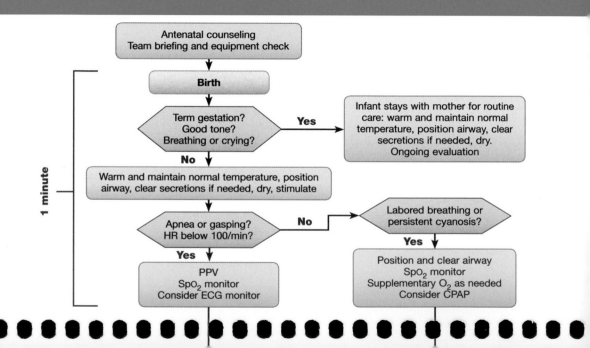

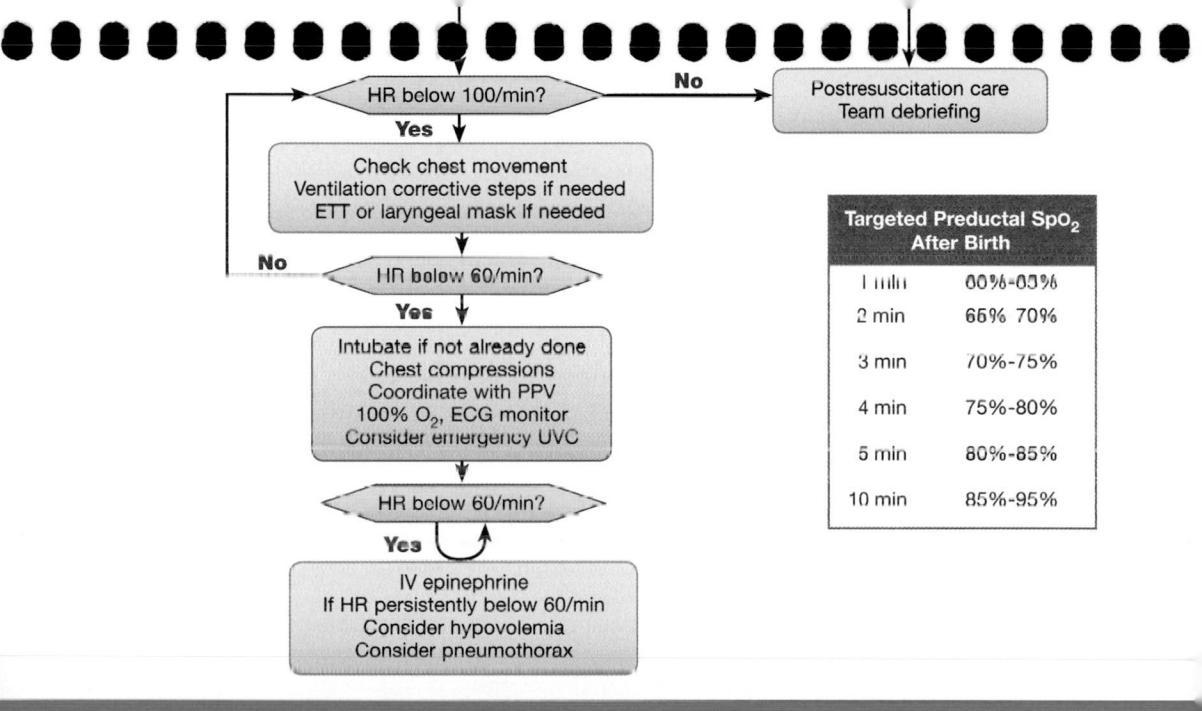

HR below 100/min? → **No** → Postresuscitation care
Team debriefing

Yes ↓

Check chest movement
Ventilation corrective steps if needed
ETT or laryngeal mask if needed

↓

No ← HR below 60/min?

Yes ↓

Intubate if not already done
Chest compressions
Coordinate with PPV
100% O_2, ECG monitor
Consider emergency UVC

↓

HR below 60/min?

Yes ↻

IV epinephrine
If HR persistently below 60/min
Consider hypovolemia
Consider pneumothorax

Targeted Preductal SpO$_2$ After Birth	
1 min	60%–65%
2 min	65% 70%
3 min	70%–75%
4 min	75%–80%
5 min	80%–85%
10 min	85%–95%

Initial Cardiopulmonary Resuscitation

Ventilation rate: 40 to 60/min when performed *without* compressions.

Compression rate: 120 events/min (90 compressions interspersed with 30 ventilations).

Compression-ventilation ratio: 3:1 (pause compressions for ventilation).

Medications (epinephrine, volume): Indicated if heart rate remains <60/min despite adequate ventilation with 100% oxygen and chest compressions.

Estimation of Proper Endotracheal Tube Size and Depth of Insertion Based on Infant's Gestational Age and Weight

Gestational Age (wk)	ETT Insertion Depth at Lips (cm)	Infant's Weight (g)
23-24	5.5	500-600
25-26	6.0	700-800
27-29	6.5	900-1000
30-32	7.0	1100-1400
33-34	7.5	1500-1800
35-37	8.0	1900-2400
38-40	8.5	2500-3100
41-43	9.0	3200-4200

Endotracheal Tube Size for Infants of Various Weights and Gestational Ages

Weight (g)	Gestational Age (wk)	ETT Size (mm) (internal diameter)
<1000	<28	2.5
1000-2000	28-34	3.0
>2000	>34	3.5

Initial endotracheal tube insertion depth ("tip to lip") for orotracheal intubation.

Adapted from Kempley ST, Moreiras JW, Petrone FL. Endotracheal tube length for neonatal intubation. *Resuscitation.* 2008;77(3):369-373. With permission from Elsevier.

Medications Used During or Following Resuscitation of the Newborn

Medications	Dose/Route*	Concentration	Wt (kg)	Total IV/IO Volume (mL)	Precautions
Epinephrine	IV/IO (UVC preferred route) 0.01–0.03 mg/kg Higher IV/IO doses not recommended Endotracheal 0.05–0.1 mg/kg	1:10 000	1 2 3 4	0.1–0.3 0.2–0.6 0.3–0.9 0.4–1.2	Give rapidly. Repeat every 3 to 5 minutes if HR <60 with compressions.
Volume expanders Isotonic crystalloid (normal saline) or blood	10 mL/kg IV/IO		1 2 3 4	10 20 30 40	Indicated for shock. Give over 5 to 10 minutes. Reassess after each bolus
Special considerations after restoring vital signs:					
Sodium bicarbonate (4.2% solution)	1 to 2 mEq/kg IV/IO	0.5 mEq/mL (4.2% solution)	1 2 3 4	2–4 4–8 6–12 8–16	Only for prolonged resuscitation. Use only if infant is effectively ventilated before administration. Give slow push, minimum 2 minutes.
Dextrose (10% solution)	0.2 g/kg, followed by 5 mL/kg per hour D$_{10}$ IV/IO infusion	0.1 g/mL	1 2 3 4	2 4 6 8	Indicated for blood glucose <40 mg/dL. Check blood glucose 20 minutes after bolus.

Abbreviations: HR, heart rate; IO, intraosseous; IV, intravascular; UVC, umbilical vein catheter; Wt, weight.

*Endotracheal dose may not result in effective plasma concentration of drug, so vascular access should be established as soon as possible. Drugs given endotracheally require higher dosing than when given IV/IO.

Use this algorithm to determine the likelihood of congenital heart disease (CHD) in the cyanotic neonate.

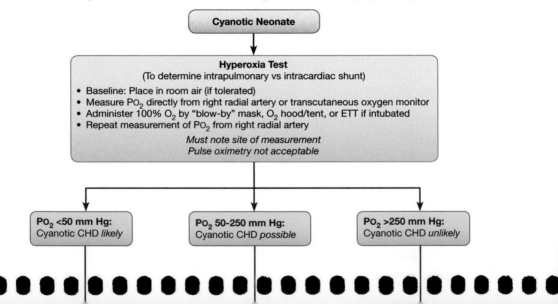

Cyanotic Neonate

Hyperoxia Test
(To determine intrapulmonary vs intracardiac shunt)

- Baseline: Place in room air (if tolerated)
- Measure PO_2 directly from right radial artery or transcutaneous oxygen monitor
- Administer 100% O_2 by "blow-by" mask, O_2 hood/tent, or ETT if intubated
- Repeat measurement of PO_2 from right radial artery

Must note site of measurement
Pulse oximetry not acceptable

PO_2 <50 mm Hg:
Cyanotic CHD *likely*

PO_2 50-250 mm Hg:
Cyanotic CHD *possible*

PO_2 >250 mm Hg:
Cyanotic CHD *unlikely*

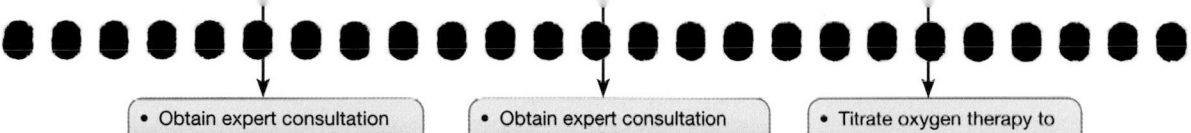

- Obtain expert consultation
- Give prostaglandin E₁ (PGE₁)

- Obtain expert consultation
- Consider PGE₁ administration

- Titrate oxygen therapy to avoid hypoxia or hyperoxia
- Avoid hypercarbia

Comparison of Differential and Reverse Differential Cyanosis
(≥10% saturation difference between right arm vs right or left leg)

	Preductal Saturation (eg, right arm)	Postductal Saturation (eg, right or left leg)	Differential Diagnosis	Initial Treatment
Differential Cyanosis	Higher	Lower	• Left-sided obstructive lesion (eg, coarctation of the aorta, interrupted aortic arch, critical aortic stenosis, hypoplastic left heart syndrome) with patent ductus arteriosus • Persistent pulmonary hypertension of the newborn with patent ductus arteriosus	• Administer prostaglandin E₁ • Obtain expert consultation
Reverse Differential Cyanosis	Lower	Higher	• Transposition of the great arteries with left-sided obstructive lesion and patent ductus arteriosus • Transposition of the great arteries with persistent pulmonary hypertension of the newborn and patent ductus arteriosus	

Pediatric Advanced Life Support

Primary cardiac arrest in children is much less common than in adults. **Cardiac arrest in children typically results from progressive deterioration in respiratory or cardiovascular function.** To prevent pediatric cardiac arrest, providers must detect and treat respiratory failure, respiratory arrest, and shock.

Conditions Indicating Need for Rapid Assessment and Potential Cardiopulmonary Support

- Irregular respirations or rate >60 breaths/min
- Heart rate ranges (particularly if associated with poor perfusion)
  - Child ≤2 years of age: <80/min or >180/min
  - Child >2 years of age: <60/min or >160/min
- Poor perfusion, with weak or absent distal pulses
- Increased work of breathing (retractions, nasal flaring, grunting)
- Cyanosis or a decrease in oxyhemoglobin saturation
- Altered level of consciousness (unusual irritability or lethargy or failure to respond to parents or painful procedures)
- Seizures
- Fever with petechiae
- Trauma
- Burns involving >10% of body surface area

Vital Signs in Children

The 3 tables below are from Hazinski MF. Children are different. In: *Nursing Care of the Critically Ill Child.* 3rd ed. St Louis, MO. Mosby; 2013:1-18, copyright Elsevier.

Normal Heart Rates*

Age	Awake Rate (beats/min)	Sleeping Rate (beats/min)
Neonate	100-205	90-160
Infant	100-180	90-160
Toddler	98-140	80-120
Preschooler	80-120	65-100
School-age child	75-110	58-90
Adolescent	60-100	50-90

*Always consider the patient's normal range and clinical condition. Heart rate will normally increase with fever or stress.

Normal Respiratory Rates*

Age	Rate (breaths/min)
Infant	30-53
Toddler	22-37
Preschooler	20-28
School-age child	18-25
Adolescent	12-20

*Consider the patient's normal range. The child's respiratory rate is expected to increase in the presence of fever or stress.
Data from Fleming S et al. *Lancet.* 2011;377(0770):1011-1018.

Normal Blood Pressures

Age	Systolic Pressure (mm Hg)*	Diastolic Pressure (mm Hg)*	Mean Arterial Pressure (mm Hg)†
Birth (12 h, <1000 g)	39-59	16-36	28-42‡
Birth (12 h, 3 kg)	60-76	31-45	48-57
Neonate (96 h)	67-84	35-53	45-60
Infant (1-12 mo)	72-104	37-56	50-62
Toddler (1-2 y)	86-106	42-63	49-62
Preschooler (3-5 y)	89-112	46-72	58-69
School-age child (6-7 y)	97-115	57-76	66-72
Preadolescent (10-12 y)	102-120	61-80	71-79
Adolescent (12-15 y)	110-131	64-83	73-84

*Systolic and diastolic blood pressure ranges assume 50th percentile for height for children 1 year and older.
†Mean arterial pressures (Diastolic pressure + [Difference between systolic and diastolic pressures ÷ 3]) for 1 year and older, assuming 50th percentile for height
‡Approximately equal to postconception age in weeks (may add 5 mm Hg).
Data from Gemelli M et al. *Eur J Pediatr.* 1990;149(5)318-320; Versmold HT et al. *Pediatrics.* 1981;67(5):607-613; Haque IU, Zaritsky AL. *Pediatr Crit Care Med.* 2007;8(2):138-144; and National Heart, Lung, and Blood Institute: *The Fourth Report on the Diagnosis, Evaluation, and Treatment of High Blood Pressure in Children and Adolescents.* NIH Publication No. 05-5267. Bethesda, MD: NHLBI; revised May 2005.

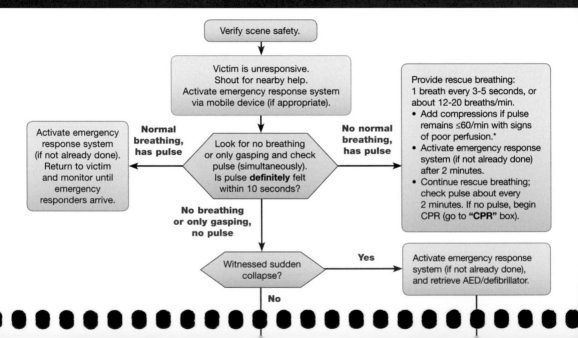

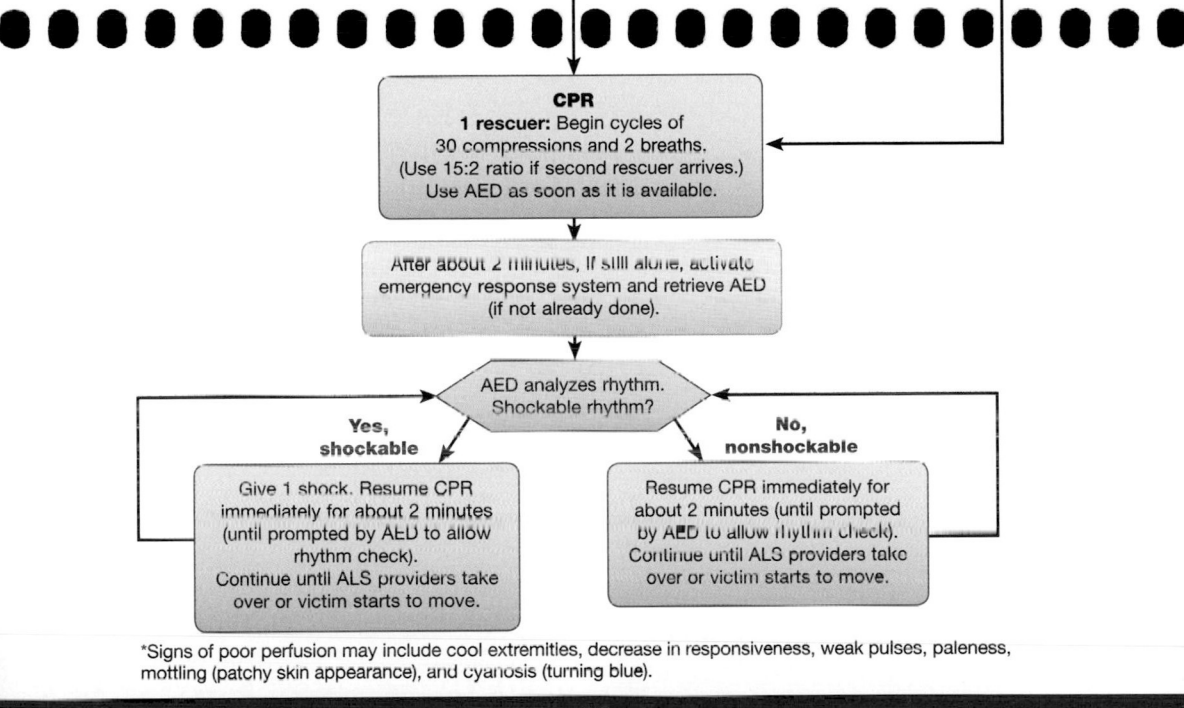

CPR
1 rescuer: Begin cycles of
30 compressions and 2 breaths.
(Use 15:2 ratio if second rescuer arrives.)
Use AED as soon as it is available.

After about 2 minutes, if still alone, activate
emergency response system and retrieve AED
(if not already done).

AED analyzes rhythm.
Shockable rhythm?

Yes,
shockable

No,
nonshockable

Give 1 shock. Resume CPR
immediately for about 2 minutes
(until prompted by AED to allow
rhythm check).
Continue until ALS providers take
over or victim starts to move.

Resume CPR immediately for
about 2 minutes (until prompted
by AED to allow rhythm check).
Continue until ALS providers take
over or victim starts to move.

*Signs of poor perfusion may include cool extremities, decrease in responsiveness, weak pulses, paleness, mottling (patchy skin appearance), and cyanosis (turning blue).

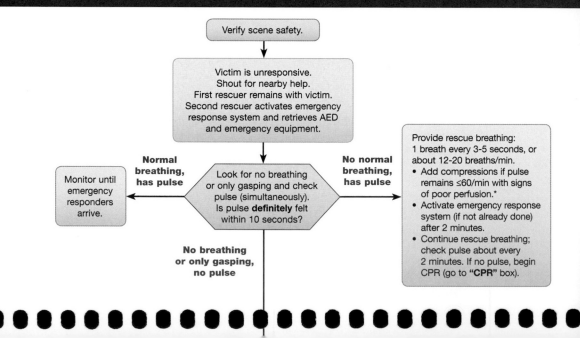

Verify scene safety.

Victim is unresponsive.
Shout for nearby help.
First rescuer remains with victim.
Second rescuer activates emergency response system and retrieves AED and emergency equipment.

Normal breathing, has pulse

Monitor until emergency responders arrive.

Look for no breathing or only gasping and check pulse (simultaneously). Is pulse **definitely** felt within 10 seconds?

No normal breathing, has pulse

Provide rescue breathing: 1 breath every 3-5 seconds, or about 12-20 breaths/min.
- Add compressions if pulse remains ≤60/min with signs of poor perfusion.*
- Activate emergency response system (if not already done) after 2 minutes.
- Continue rescue breathing; check pulse about every 2 minutes. If no pulse, begin CPR (go to **"CPR"** box).

No breathing or only gasping, no pulse

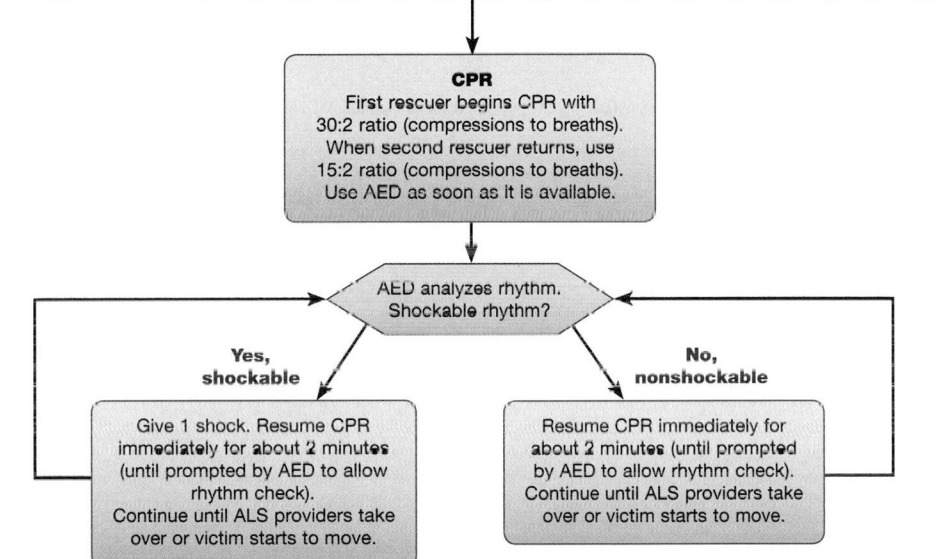

CPR
First rescuer begins CPR with
30:2 ratio (compressions to breaths).
When second rescuer returns, use
15:2 ratio (compressions to breaths).
Use AED as soon as it is available.

AED analyzes rhythm.
Shockable rhythm?

Yes,
shockable

No,
nonshockable

Give 1 shock. Resume CPR
immediately for about 2 minutes
(until prompted by AED to allow
rhythm check).
Continue until ALS providers take
over or victim starts to move.

Resume CPR immediately for
about 2 minutes (until prompted
by AED to allow rhythm check).
Continue until ALS providers take
over or victim starts to move.

*Signs of poor perfusion may include cool extremities, decrease in responsiveness, weak pulses, paleness, mottling (patchy skin appearance), and cyanosis (turning blue).

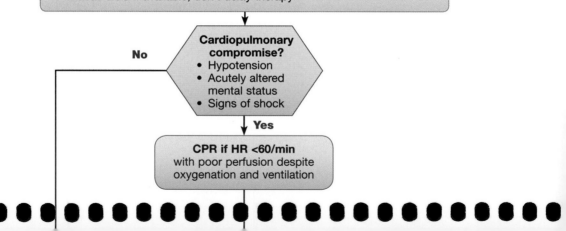

Identify and treat underlying cause

- Maintain patent airway; assist breathing as necessary
- Oxygen
- Cardiac monitor to identify rhythm; monitor blood pressure and oximetry
- IO/IV access
- 12-Lead ECG if available; don't delay therapy

No

Cardiopulmonary compromise?
- Hypotension
- Acutely altered mental status
- Signs of shock

Yes

CPR if HR <60/min
with poor perfusion despite oxygenation and ventilation

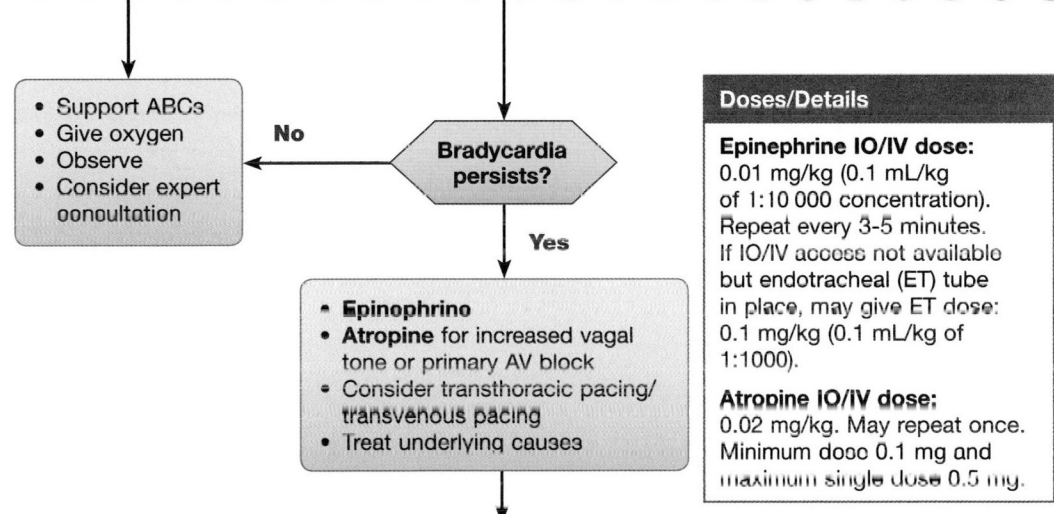

- Support ABCs
- Give oxygen
- Observe
- Consider expert consultation

No

Bradycardia persists?

Yes

- **Epinephrine**
- **Atropine** for increased vagal tone or primary AV block
- Consider transthoracic pacing/ transvenous pacing
- Treat underlying causes

Doses/Details

Epinephrine IO/IV dose:
0.01 mg/kg (0.1 mL/kg of 1:10 000 concentration). Repeat every 3-5 minutes. If IO/IV access not available but endotracheal (ET) tube in place, may give ET dose: 0.1 mg/kg (0.1 mL/kg of 1:1000).

Atropine IO/IV dose:
0.02 mg/kg. May repeat once. Minimum dose 0.1 mg and maximum single dose 0.5 mg.

If pulseless arrest develops, go to Cardiac Arrest Algorithm

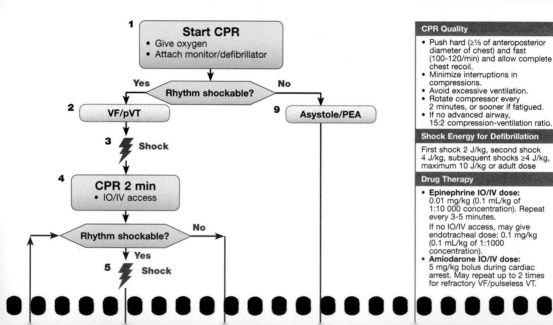

CPR Quality

- Push hard (≥⅓ of anteroposterior diameter of chest) and fast (100-120/min) and allow complete chest recoil.
- Minimize interruptions in compressions.
- Avoid excessive ventilation.
- Rotate compressor every 2 minutes, or sooner if fatigued.
- If no advanced airway, 15:2 compression-ventilation ratio.

Shock Energy for Defibrillation

First shock 2 J/kg, second shock 4 J/kg, subsequent shocks ≥4 J/kg, maximum 10 J/kg or adult dose

Drug Therapy

- **Epinephrine IO/IV dose:** 0.01 mg/kg (0.1 mL/kg of 1:10 000 concentration). Repeat every 3-5 minutes.
  If no IO/IV access, may give endotracheal dose: 0.1 mg/kg (0.1 mL/kg of 1:1000 concentration).
- **Amiodarone IO/IV dose:** 5 mg/kg bolus during cardiac arrest. May repeat up to 2 times for refractory VF/pulseless VT.

1 Start CPR
- Give oxygen
- Attach monitor/defibrillator

Rhythm shockable?
Yes / No

2 VF/pVT

9 Asystole/PEA

3 Shock

4 CPR 2 min
- IO/IV access

Rhythm shockable?
No / Yes

5 Shock

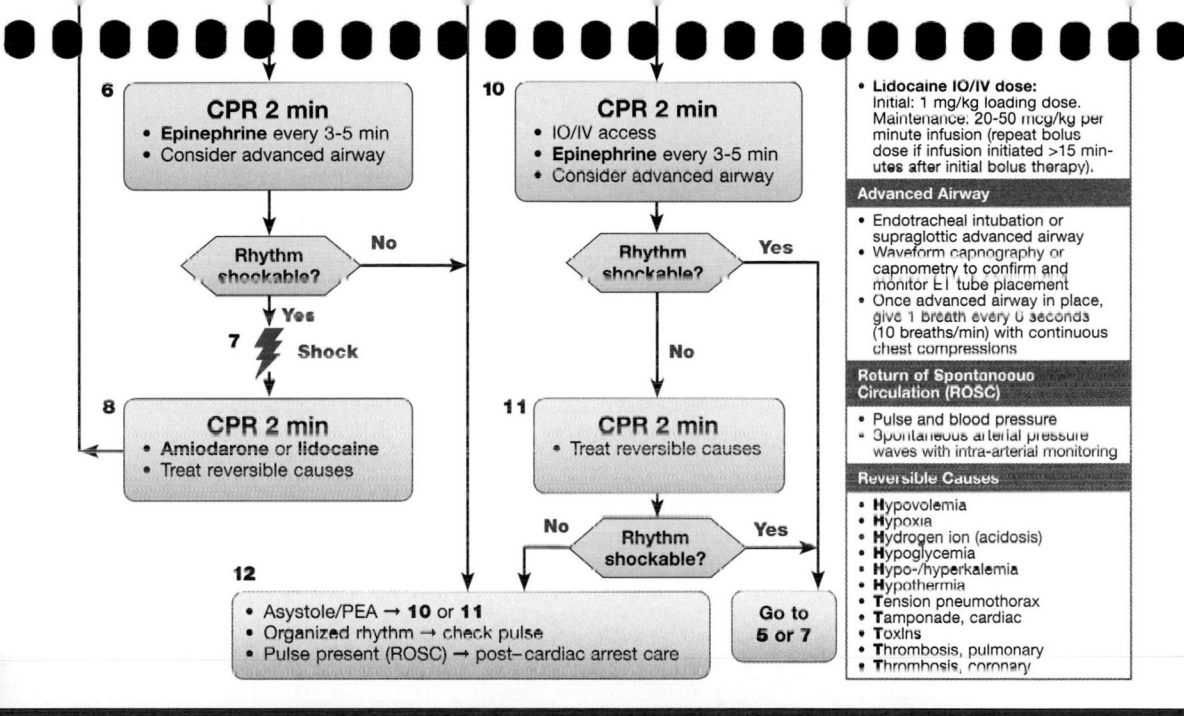

6

CPR 2 min
- **Epinephrine** every 3-5 min
- Consider advanced airway

Rhythm shockable? — No →

Yes ↓

7 ⚡ **Shock**

8

CPR 2 min
- **Amiodarone or lidocaine**
- Treat reversible causes

10

CPR 2 min
- IO/IV access
- **Epinephrine** every 3-5 min
- Consider advanced airway

Rhythm shockable? — Yes →

No ↓

11

CPR 2 min
- Treat reversible causes

No — **Rhythm shockable?** — Yes →

12
- Asystole/PEA → **10** or **11**
- Organized rhythm → check pulse
- Pulse present (ROSC) → post–cardiac arrest care

Go to 5 or 7

- **Lidocaine IO/IV dose:**
  Initial: 1 mg/kg loading dose.
  Maintenance: 20-50 mcg/kg per minute infusion (repeat bolus dose if infusion initiated >15 minutes after initial bolus therapy).

Advanced Airway
- Endotracheal intubation or supraglottic advanced airway
- Waveform capnography or capnometry to confirm and monitor ET tube placement
- Once advanced airway in place, give 1 breath every 6 seconds (10 breaths/min) with continuous chest compressions

Return of Spontaneous Circulation (ROSC)
- Pulse and blood pressure
- Spontaneous arterial pressure waves with intra-arterial monitoring

Reversible Causes
- **H**ypovolemia
- **H**ypoxia
- **H**ydrogen ion (acidosis)
- **H**ypoglycemia
- **H**ypo-/hyperkalemia
- **H**ypothermia
- **T**ension pneumothorax
- **T**amponade, cardiac
- **T**oxins
- **T**hrombosis, pulmonary
- **T**hrombosis, coronary

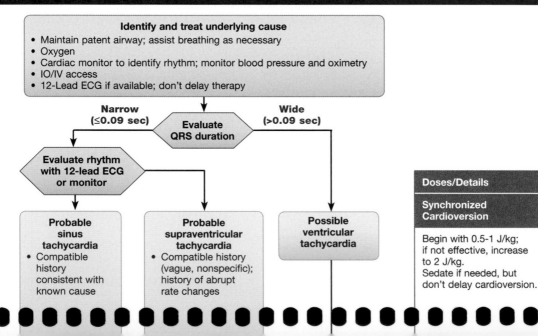

Identify and treat underlying cause
- Maintain patent airway; assist breathing as necessary
- Oxygen
- Cardiac monitor to identify rhythm; monitor blood pressure and oximetry
- IO/IV access
- 12-Lead ECG if available; don't delay therapy

Evaluate QRS duration

Narrow (≤0.09 sec)

Wide (>0.09 sec)

Evaluate rhythm with 12-lead ECG or monitor

Probable sinus tachycardia
- Compatible history consistent with known cause

Probable supraventricular tachycardia
- Compatible history (vague, nonspecific); history of abrupt rate changes

Possible ventricular tachycardia

Doses/Details
Synchronized Cardioversion
Begin with 0.5-1 J/kg; if not effective, increase to 2 J/kg. Sedate if needed, but don't delay cardioversion.

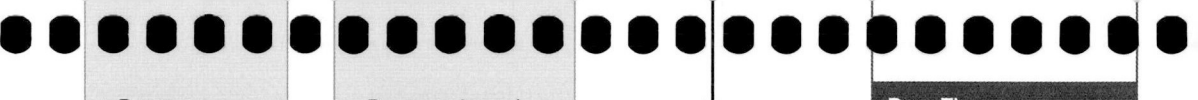

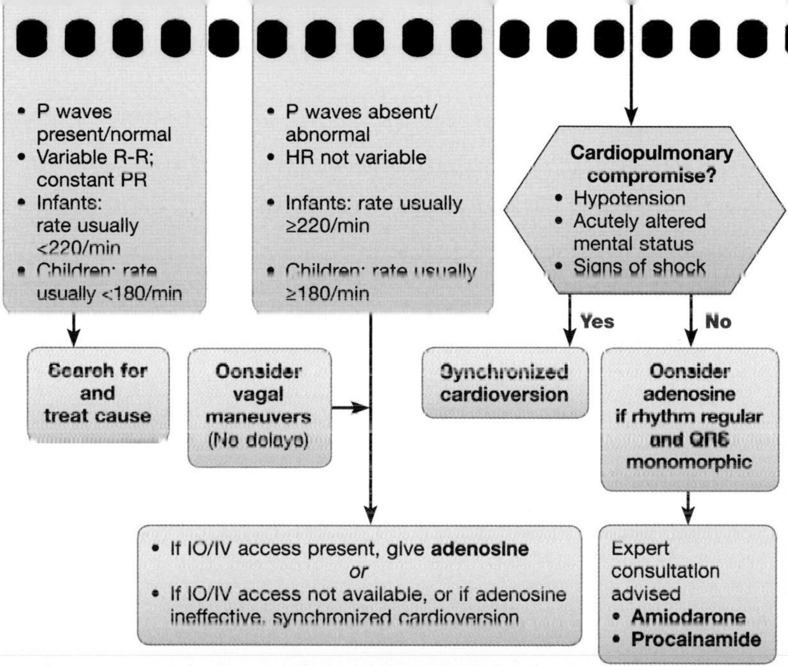

- P waves present/normal
- Variable R-R; constant PR
- Infants: rate usually <220/min
- Children: rate usually <180/min

- P waves absent/abnormal
- HR not variable
- Infants: rate usually ≥220/min
- Children: rate usually ≥180/min

Cardiopulmonary compromise?
- Hypotension
- Acutely altered mental status
- Signs of shock

Yes   **No**

Search for and treat cause

Consider vagal maneuvers (No delays)

Synchronized cardioversion

Consider adenosine if rhythm regular and QRS monomorphic

- If IO/IV access present, give **adenosine**
  or
- If IO/IV access not available, or if adenosine ineffective, synchronized cardioversion

Expert consultation advised
- **Amiodarone**
- **Procainamide**

Drug Therapy

Adenosine IO/IV dose:
First dose:
0.1 mg/kg rapid bolus (maximum: 6 mg).
Second dose:
0.2 mg/kg rapid bolus (maximum second dose: 12 mg).

Amiodarone IO/IV dose:
5 mg/kg over 20-60 minutes
or
Procainamide IO/IV dose:
15 mg/kg over 30-60 minutes

Do not routinely administer amiodarone and procainamide together.

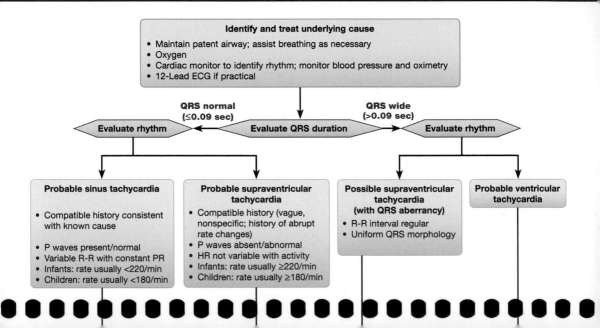

Identify and treat underlying cause

- Maintain patent airway; assist breathing as necessary
- Oxygen
- Cardiac monitor to identify rhythm; monitor blood pressure and oximetry
- 12-Lead ECG if practical

QRS normal (≤0.09 sec)

Evaluate rhythm

Evaluate QRS duration

QRS wide (>0.09 sec)

Evaluate rhythm

Probable sinus tachycardia

- Compatible history consistent with known cause

- P waves present/normal
- Variable R-R with constant PR
- Infants: rate usually <220/min
- Children: rate usually <180/min

Probable supraventricular tachycardia

- Compatible history (vague, nonspecific; history of abrupt rate changes)
- P waves absent/abnormal
- HR not variable with activity
- Infants: rate usually ≥220/min
- Children: rate usually ≥180/min

Possible supraventricular tachycardia (with QRS aberrancy)

- R-R interval regular
- Uniform QRS morphology

Probable ventricular tachycardia

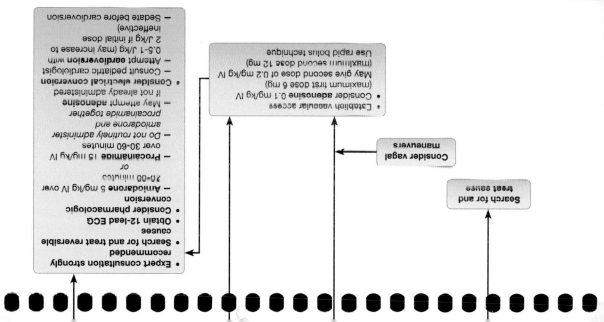

Search for and treat cause

Consider vagal maneuvers

- Establish vascular access
- Consider adenosine 0.1 mg/kg IV
  (maximum first dose 6 mg)
  May give second dose of 0.2 mg/kg IV
  (maximum second dose 12 mg)
  Use rapid bolus technique

- **Expert consultation strongly recommended**
- Search for and treat reversible causes
- Obtain 12-lead ECG
- Consider pharmacologic conversion
  — **Amiodarone 5 mg/kg IV** over 20-60 minutes
    or
  — **Procainamide 15 mg/kg IV** over 30-60 minutes
  — *Do not routinely administer amiodarone and procainamide together*
  — May attempt **adenosine** if not already administered
- Consider electrical conversion
  — Consult pediatric cardiologist
  — **Attempt cardioversion** with 0.5-1 J/kg (may increase to 2 J/kg if initial dose ineffective)
  — Sedate before cardioversion

Manual Defibrillation
(for VF or pulseless VT)

Continue CPR without interruptions during all steps until step 8. Minimize interval from compressions to shock delivery (do not deliver breaths between compressions and shock delivery).

1. Turn on defibrillator.
2. Set *lead switch* to *paddles* (or *lead I, II,* or *III* if monitor leads are used).
3. Select adhesive pads or paddles. Use the largest pads or paddles that can fit on the patient's chest without touching each other.
4. If using paddles, apply conductive gel or paste. Be sure cables are attached to defibrillator.
5. Position adhesive pads on patient's chest: right anterior chest wall and left axillary positions (or as is illustrated on pads). If using paddles, apply firm pressure. If patient has an implanted pacemaker, do not position pads/paddles directly over the device. Be sure that oxygen is not directed over patient's chest.

Cardioversion
(for unstable SVT or VT with a pulse)

Consider expert consultation for suspected VT.

1. Turn on defibrillator.
2. Set *lead switch* to *paddles* (or *lead I, II,* or *III* if monitor leads are used).
3. Select adhesive pads to paddles. Use the largest pads or paddles that can fit on the patient's chest without touching each other.
4. If using paddles, apply conductive gel or paste. Be sure cables are attached to defibrillator.
5. Consider sedation.
6. Select *synchronized* mode.
7. Look for markers on R waves indicating that *sync* mode is operative. If necessary, adjust monitor gain until sync markers occur with each R wave.
8. Select energy dose:
   Initial dose: 0.5-1 J/kg
   Subsequent doses: 2 J/kg

6. Select energy dose:
   Initial dose: 2 J/kg (acceptable range 2-4 J/kg)
   Subsequent doses: 4 J/kg or higher (not to
   exceed 10 J/kg or standard adult dose)

7. Announce "Charging defibrillator," and press *charge*
   on defibrillator controls or apex paddle.

8. When defibrillator is fully charged, state firm chant,
   such as
   "I am going to shock on three." Then count.
   "I am clear to shock!"
   (Chest compressions should continue until this
   announcement.)

9. After confirming all personnel are clear of the patient,
   press the *shock* button on the defibrillator or press
   the 2 paddle *discharge* buttons simultaneously.

10. Immediately after shock delivery, resume CPR
    beginning with compressions for about 5 cycles
    (about 2 minutes), and then recheck rhythm.
    Interruption of CPR should be brief.

9. Announce "Charging defibrillator," and press
   charge on defibrillator controls or apex paddle.

10. When defibrillator is fully charged, state firm
    chant, such as
    "I am going to shock on three." Then count.
    "I am clear to shock!"

11. After confirming all personnel are clear of the
    patient, press the *shock* button on the defibrillator
    or press the 2 paddle *discharge* buttons
    simultaneously. Hold paddles in place until shock
    is delivered.

12. Check the monitor. If tachycardia persists,
    increase energy and prepare to cardiovert again.

13. Reset the *sync* mode after each synchronized
    cardioversion, because most defibrillators default
    back to unsynchronized mode. This default
    allows an immediate shock if the cardioversion
    produces VF

Note: If VF develops, immediately begin CPR and
prepare to deliver an unsynchronized shock (see
Manual Defibrillation on left).

Management of Respiratory Emergencies Flowchart
• Airway positioning • Suction as needed • Oxygen • Pulse oximetry • ECG monitor (as indicated) • BLS as indicated

Upper Airway Obstruction
Specific Management for Selected Conditions

Croup	*Anaphylaxis*	*Aspiration Foreign Body*
• Nebulized epinephrine • Corticosteroids	• IM epinephrine (or auto-injector) • Albuterol • Antihistamines • Corticosteroids	• Allow position of comfort • Specialty consultation

Lower Airway Obstruction
Specific Management for Selected Conditions

Bronchiolitis	*Asthma*	
• Nasal suctioning • Bronchodilator trial	• Albuterol ± ipratropium • Corticosteroids • Subcutaneous epinephrine	• Magnesium sulfate • Terbutaline

Lung Tissue (Parenchymal) Disease
Specific Management for Selected Conditions

Pneumonia/Pneumonitis *Infectious Chemical Aspiration*	*Pulmonary Edema* *Cardiogenic or Noncardiogenic (ARDS)*
• Albuterol • Antibiotics (as indicated) • Consider CPAP	• Consider noninvasive or invasive ventilatory support with PEEP • Consider vasoactive support • Consider diuretic

Disordered Control of Breathing
Specific Management for Selected Conditions

Increased ICP	*Poisoning/Overdose*	*Neuromuscular Disease*
• Avoid hypoxemia • Avoid hypercarbia • Avoid hyperthermia	• Antidote (if available) • Contact poison control	• Consider noninvasive or invasive ventilatory support

Pre-event Equipment Checklist for Endotracheal Intubation

☐	Universal precautions (gloves, mask, eye protection)
☐	Cardiac monitor, pulse oximeter, and blood pressure monitoring device
☐	End-tidal CO_2 detector or exhaled CO_2 capnography
☐	Intravenous and intraosseous infusion equipment
☐	Oxygen supply, bag-mask (appropriate size)
☐	Oral/tracheal suction equipment (appropriate size); confirm that it is working
☐	Oral and nasopharyngeal airways (appropriate size)
☐	Endotracheal tubes with stylets (all sizes, with and without cuffs) and sizes 0.5 mm (i.d.) above and below anticipated size for patient
☐	Laryngoscope (curved and straight blades) and/or video laryngoscope; backup laryngoscope available
☐	3-, 5-, and 10-mL syringes to test inflate endotracheal tube balloon
☐	Cuff pressure monitor (if using cuffed tubes)
☐	Adhesive/cloth tape or commercial endotracheal tube holder to secure tube
☐	Towel or pad to align airway by placing under head or torso
☐	Specialty equipment as needed for difficult airway management or anticipated complications (supraglottic, transtracheal, and/or cricothyrotomy)

RSI Protocol for PALS

Pre-event preparation	1. Obtain brief medical history and perform focused physical examination.
	2. Prepare equipment, monitors, personnel, medications.
	3. If neck injury not suspected: place in sniffing position.
	If neck injury suspected: stabilize cervical spine.
Preoxygenate	4. Preoxygenate with Fio_2 of 100% by mask (nonrebreather preferred). If ventilatory assistance is necessary, ventilate gently.
Premedicate/sedate	5. Premedicate and sedate as appropriate; wait briefly to allow adequate sedation after drug administration.
Pharmacologic sedation/anesthesia/ neuromuscular blockade and protection/positioning	6. Administer sedation/anesthesia by IV push.
	7. Give neuromuscular blocking agent by IV push
	8. Apply cricoid pressure.
	9. Assess for apnea, jaw relaxation, and absence of movement (patient sufficiently relaxed to proceed with intubation).
Placement of endotracheal tube	10. Perform endotracheal intubation. If during intubation oxygen saturation is inadequate, stop laryngoscopy and start ventilation with bag-mask. Monitor pulse oximetry and ensure adequate oxygen saturation. Reattempt intubation. Once intubated, inflate cuff (if cuffed tracheal tube is used) to minimal occlusive volume. Be prepared to place rescue airway if intubation attempts are unsuccessful.
Placement confirmation	11. Confirm placement of endotracheal tube by • direct visualization of ET passing through vocal cords • chest rise/fall with each ventilation (bilateral) • 5-point auscultation: anterior chest L and R, midaxillary line L and R, and over the epigastrium (no breath sounds over epigastrium); look for tube condensation • using end tidal CO_2 meter (or esophageal detector device, if appropriate) • monitoring O_2 saturation and exhaled CO_2 levels (capnometry or waveform capnography)
Postintubation management	12. Prevent dislodgement: • Secure ET with adhesive/cloth tape or commercial ET holder • Continue cervical spine immobilization (if needed) • Continue sedation; add paralytics if necessary • Check cuff inflation pressure

Pharmacologic Agents Used for Rapid Sequence Intubation in Children

Drug	IV/IO Dose*	Onset	Duration	Side Effects	Comments
Premedication Agents					
Atropine	0.01-0.02 mg/kg (maximum: 0.5 mg)	1-2 min	2-4 hours	Tachycardia, agitation	Antisialogogue Inhibits bradycardic response to hypoxia, laryngoscopy, and succinylcholine May cause pupil dilation
Glycopyrrolate	0.005-0.01 mg/kg (maximum: 0.2 mg)	1-2 min	4-6 hours	Tachycardia	Antisialogogue Inhibits bradycardic response to hypoxia
Lidocaine	1-2 mg/kg	1-2 min	10-20 min	Myocardial and CNS depression with high doses Seizures	May decrease ICP during RSI May decrease pain on propofol injection
Sedative Agents					
Etomidate	0.2-0.4 mg/kg	<1 min	5-10 min	Myoclonic activity Cortisol suppression	Ultrashort acting No analgesic properties Decreases cerebral metabolic rate and ICP Generally maintains hemodynamic stability Avoid routine use in patients with suspected septic shock

| Fentanyl citrate | 2-5 mcg/kg | 1-3 min | 30-60 min | Chest wall rigidity possible with high-dose rapid infusions | Minimum histamine release
May lower blood pressure (especially with higher doses or in conjunction with midazolam) |
|---|---|---|---|---|---|
| Ketamine | 1-2 mg/kg | 30-60 sec | 10-20 min | Hypertension, tachycardia
Increased secretions and laryngospasm
Emergence reactions/ hallucinations | Dissociative anesthetic agent
Limited respiratory depression
Bronchodilator
May cause myocardial depression in catecholamine-depleted patients
Use with caution in patients with potential or increased ICP |
| Midazolam | 0.1-0.3 mg/kg (maximum single dose: 10 mg) | 2-5 min | 15-30 min | Hypotension | Hypotension exacerbated in combination with narcotics and barbiturates
No analgesic properties
Excellent amnesia |
| Diazepam | 0.2-0.3 mg/kg (maximum single dose: 10 mg) | 1-3 min | 20-40 min | | |

Abbreviations: CNS, central nervous system; ICP, intracranial pressure; IO, intraosseous; IV, intravascular; RSI, rapid sequence intubation.

*Doses provided are guidelines only. Actual dosing may vary depending on patient's clinical status

(continued)

Pharmacologic Agents Used for Rapid Sequence Intubation in Children *(continued)*

Drug	IV/IO Dose*	Onset	Duration	Side Effects	Comments
Sedative Agents *(continued)*					
Propofol	1-2 mg/kg (up to 3 mg/kg in children 6 months to 5 years of age)	<1 min	5-10 min	Hypotension, especially in patients with inadequate intravascular volume Pain on infusion	No analgesic properties Very short duration of action Less airway reactivity than barbiturates Decreases cerebral metabolic rate and ICP Lidocaine may decrease infusion pain Not recommended in patients with egg/soy allergy

Drug	IV/IO Dose*	Time to Paralysis	Duration of Paralysis	Side Effects	Comments
Neuromuscular Blocking Agents					
Succinylcholine	1-1.5 mg/kg for children; 2 mg/kg for infants	45-60 sec	4-6 min	May cause rhabdomyolysis; rise in intracranial, intraocular, intragastric pressure; life-threatening hyperkalemia	Depolarizing muscle relaxant Rapid onset, short duration of action Avoid in renal failure, burns, crush injuries after 48 hours, muscular dystrophy and other neuromuscular diseases, hyperkalemia, or family history of malignant hyperthermia Do *not* use to maintain paralysis
Vecuronium	0.1-0.3 mg/kg	1-3 min	30-60 min	Minimal cardiovascular side effects	Nondepolarizing agent The higher the dose, the quicker the onset of action and the longer the duration
Rocuronium	0.6-1.2 mg/kg	30-60 sec	30-60 min	Minimal cardiovascular side effects	Nondepolarizing agent Rapid onset of action

Abbreviations: ICP, intracranial pressure; IO, intraosseous; IV, intravenous

*Doses provided are guidelines only. Actual dosing may vary depending on patient's clinical status.

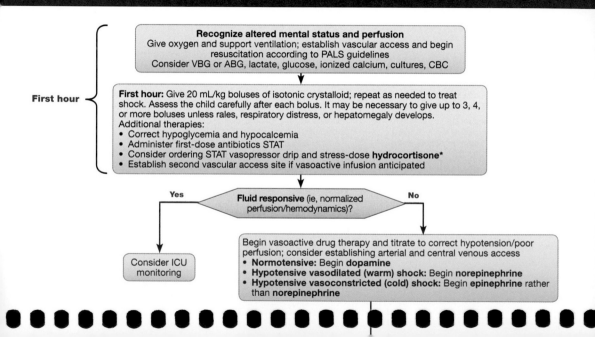

First hour

Recognize altered mental status and perfusion
Give oxygen and support ventilation; establish vascular access and begin resuscitation according to PALS guidelines
Consider VBG or ABG, lactate, glucose, ionized calcium, cultures, CBC

First hour: Give 20 mL/kg boluses of isotonic crystalloid; repeat as needed to treat shock. Assess the child carefully after each bolus. It may be necessary to give up to 3, 4, or more boluses unless rales, respiratory distress, or hepatomegaly develops.
Additional therapies:
- Correct hypoglycemia and hypocalcemia
- Administer first-dose antibiotics STAT
- Consider ordering STAT vasopressor drip and stress-dose **hydrocortisone***
- Establish second vascular access site if vasoactive infusion anticipated

Fluid responsive (ie, normalized perfusion/hemodynamics)?

Yes

No

Consider ICU monitoring

Begin vasoactive drug therapy and titrate to correct hypotension/poor perfusion; consider establishing arterial and central venous access
- **Normotensive:** Begin **dopamine**
- **Hypotensive vasodilated (warm) shock:** Begin **norepinephrine**
- **Hypotensive vasoconstricted (cold) shock:** Begin **epinephrine** rather than **norepinephrine**

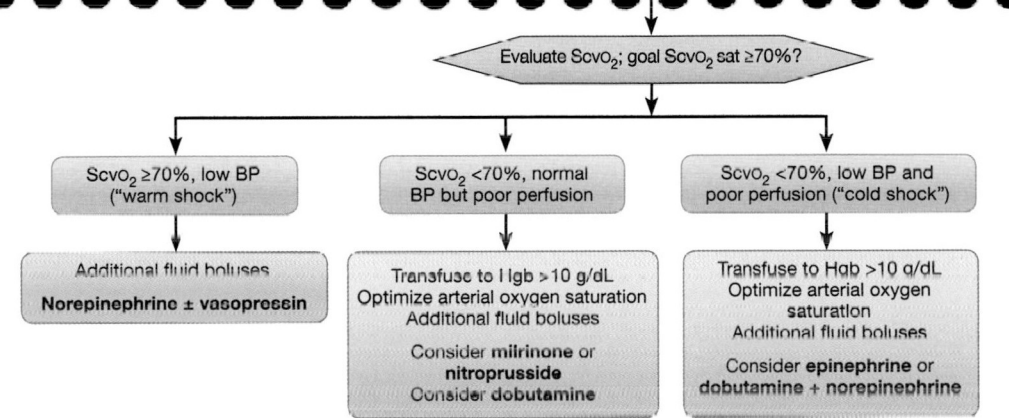

Evaluate Scvo₂; goal Scvo₂ sat ≥70%?

Scvo₂ ≥70%, low BP ("warm shock")	Scvo₂ <70%, normal BP but poor perfusion	Scvo₂ <70%, low BP and poor perfusion ("cold shock")
Additional fluid boluses **Norepinephrine ± vasopressin**	Transfuse to Hgb >10 g/dL Optimize arterial oxygen saturation Additional fluid boluses Consider **milrinone** or **nitroprusside** Consider **dobutamine**	Transfuse to Hgb >10 g/dL Optimize arterial oxygen saturation Additional fluid boluses Consider **epinephrine** or **dobutamine + norepinephrine**

*Fluid-refractory and dopamine- or norepinephrine-dependent shock defines patient at risk for adrenal insufficiency.

If adrenal insufficiency is suspected give **hydrocortisone** ~2 mg/kg bolus IV; maximum 100 mg

Draw baseline cortisol; consider ACTH stimulation test if unsure of need for steroids

Modified from Brierley J, Carcillo JA, Choong K, et al. Clinical practice parameters for hemodynamic support of pediatric and neonatal septic shock: 2007 update from the American College of Critical Care Medicine. *Crit Care Med.* 2009;37(2):666-688.

Glasgow Coma Scale for Adults* and Modified Glasgow Coma Scale for Infants and Children†

Response	Adult	Child	Infant	Coded Value
Eye opening	Spontaneous	Spontaneous	Spontaneous	4
	To speech	To speech	To speech	3
	To pain	To pain	To pain	2
	None	None	None	1
Best verbal response	Oriented	Oriented, appropriate	Coos and babbles	5
	Confused	Confused	Irritable, cries	4
	Inappropriate words	Inappropriate words	Cries in response to pain	3
	Incomprehensible sounds	Incomprehensible words or nonspecific sounds	Moans in response to pain	2
	None	None	None	1

Best motor response[†]	Obeys	Obeys commands	Moves spontaneously and purposely	6
	Localizes	Localizes painful stimulus	Withdraws in response to touch	5
	Withdraws	Withdraws in response to pain	Withdraws in response to pain	4
	Abnormal flexion	Flexion in response to pain	Decorticate posturing (abnormal flexion) in response to pain	3
	Extensor response	Extension in response to pain	Decerebrate posturing (abnormal extension) in response to pain	2
	None	None	None	1
Total score				**3-15**

*Teasdale G, Jennett B. Assessment of coma and impaired consciousness: a practical scale. *Lancet.* 1974;2(7872):81-84.

†Modified from James HE, Trauner DA. The Glasgow Coma Scale. In: James HE, Anas NG, Perkin RM, eds. *Brain Insults in Infants and Children: Pathophysiology and Management.* Orlando, FL: Grune & Stratton; 1985:179-182; and Hazinski MF. Neurologic disorders. In: Hazinski MF. *Nursing Care of the Critically Ill Child.* 2nd ed. St Louis, MO: Mosby-Year Book; 1992:521-628, copyright Elsevier.

‡If the patient is intubated, unconscious, or preverbal, the most important part of this scale is motor response. Providers should carefully evaluate this component.

System	Mild Blood Volume Loss (<30%)	Moderate Blood Volume Loss (30%-45%)	Severe Blood Volume Loss (>45%)
Cardiovascular	Increased heart rate; weak, thready peripheral pulses; normal systolic blood pressure (80-90 + 2 × age in years); normal pulse pressure	Markedly increased heart rate; weak, thready central pulses; absent peripheral pulses; low normal systolic blood pressure (70-80 + 2 × age in years); narrowed pulse pressure	Tachycardia followed by bradycardia; very weak or absent peripheral pulses; hypotension (<70 + 2 × age in years); undetectable diastolic blood pressure (or widened pulse pressure)
Central nervous system	Anxious; irritable; confused	Lethargic; dulled response to pain*	Comatose
Skin	Cool, mottled; prolonged capillary refill	Cyanotic; markedly prolonged capillary refill	Pale and cold
Urine output†	Low to very low	Minimal	None

*The child's dulled response to pain with this degree of blood loss (30%-45%) may be indicated by a decreased response to IV catheter insertion.

†After initial decompression by urinary catheter. Low normal is 2 mL/kg per hour (infant), 1.5 mL/kg per hour (younger child), 1 mL/kg per hour (older child), and 0.5 mL/kg per hour (adolescent). Intravenous contrast can falsely elevate urinary output.

Adaptation of the original table from American College of Surgeons. *Advanced Trauma Life Support® Student Course Manual.* 9th ed. Chicago, IL: American College of Surgeons; 2012.

Approach to Fluid Resuscitation in Child With Multiple Injuries

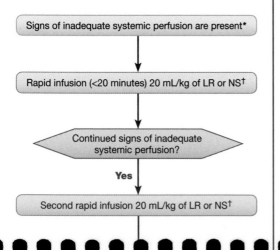

Signs of inadequate systemic perfusion are present*

↓

Rapid infusion (<20 minutes) 20 mL/kg of LR or NS†

↓

Continued signs of inadequate systemic perfusion?

Yes

↓

Second rapid infusion 20 mL/kg of LR or NS†

Approach to the Child With Multiple Injuries

Effective trauma resuscitation requires a team effort. The assessments and interventions below may be performed simultaneously. Initiate CPR when needed.

1. Before arrival, notify trauma surgeon with pediatric expertise.

2. Open airway with jaw thrust, maintaining manual cervical spine stabilization.

3. Clear the oropharynx with a rigid suction device; assess breathing.

4. Administer 100% oxygen by nonrebreathing mask if child is responsive and breathing spontaneously.

5. Ventilate with bag-mask device and 100% oxygen if child has inadequate respiratory effort or respiratory distress or is unresponsive. Hyperventilate only if there are signs of impending brain herniation.

6. Provide advanced airway management with appropriate manual cervical spine stabilization if the child has signs of respiratory failure or is unresponsive. Trained healthcare providers may attempt endotracheal intubation; confirm endotracheal tube placement with clinical assessment and a device (eg, exhaled CO_2 detector, esophageal detector device). If the child is unconscious during bag-mask ventilation, consider use of an oropharyngeal airway and cricoid pressure.

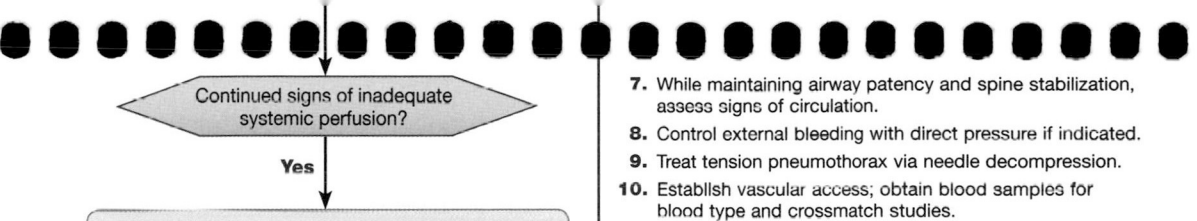

Continued signs of inadequate
systemic perfusion?

Yes

- Third rapid infusion 20 mL/kg of LR or NS†

    or

- Packed RBCs (10 mL/kg), mixed with NS, bolus

    Repeat every 20 to 30 minutes, as needed

7. While maintaining airway patency and spine stabilization, assess signs of circulation.

8. Control external bleeding with direct pressure if indicated.

9. Treat tension pneumothorax via needle decompression.

10. Establish vascular access; obtain blood samples for blood type and crossmatch studies.

11. Rapidly infuse 20 mL/kg isotonic crystalloid for inadequate perfusion.

12. Immobilize the neck with a semirigid collar, head immobilizer, and tape. In prehospital settings, immobilize thighs, pelvis, shoulders, and head to long spine board.

13. Consider gastric decompression (an orogastric tube is preferred if head trauma is present).

14. Infuse a second isotonic crystalloid bolus if signs of shock are present. Consider blood products for major hemorrhage.

15. Consider need for surgical exploration if hypotension is present on arrival or if hemodynamic instability persists despite crystalloid and blood administration.

*In child with severe trauma and life-threatening blood loss:
- Blood for STAT type and crossmatch; type specific blood is preferred, time permitting
- Use O-negative blood in females and O-positive or O-negative blood in males when possible

†If LR is not available, NS may be used.

Management of Shock After ROSC

Optimize Ventilation and Oxygenation
- Titrate FIO_2 to maintain oxyhemoglobin saturation 94%-99% (or as appropriate to the patient's condition); if possible, wean FIO_2 if saturation is 100%.
- Consider advanced airway placement and waveform capnography.
- If possible, target a PCO_2 that is appropriate for the patient's condition and limit exposure to severe hypercapnia or hypocapnia.

↓

Assess for and Treat Persistent Shock
- Identify and treat contributing factors.*
- Consider 20 mL/kg IV/IO boluses of isotonic crystalloid. Consider smaller boluses (eg, 10 mL/kg) if poor cardiac function suspected.
- Consider the need for inotropic and/or vasopressor support for fluid-refractory shock.

↔

*Possible Contributing Factors
Hypovolemia
Hypoxia
Hydrogen ion (acidosis)
Hypoglycemia
Hypo-/hyperkalemia
Hypothermia
Tension pneumothorax
Tamponade, cardiac
Toxins
Thrombosis, pulmonary
Thrombosis, coronary
Trauma

Estimation of Maintenance Fluid Requirements

- **Infants <10 kg:** 4 mL/kg per hour

  Example: For an 8-kg infant, estimated maintenance fluid rate
  = 4 mL/kg per hour × 8 kg
  = 32 mL per hour

- **Children 10-20 kg:** 4 mL/kg per hour for the first 10 kg + 2 mL/kg per hour for each kg above 10 kg

  Example: For a 15-kg child, estimated maintenance fluid rate
  = (4 mL/kg per hour × 10 kg)
  + (2 mL/kg per hour × 5 kg)
  = 40 mL/hour + 10 mL/hour
  = 50 mL/hour

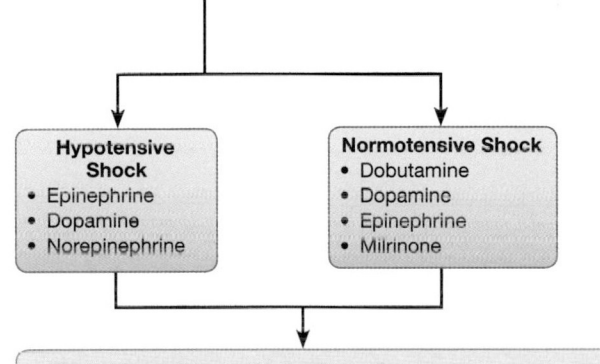

Hypotensive Shock
- Epinephrine
- Dopamine
- Norepinephrine

Normotensive Shock
- Dobutamine
- Dopamine
- Epinephrine
- Milrinone

- Monitor for and treat agitation and seizures.
- Monitor for and treat hypoglycemia.
- Assess blood gas, serum electrolytes, and calcium.
- If patient remains comatose after resuscitation from cardiac arrest, maintain targeted temperature management, including aggressive treatment of fever.
- Consider consultation and patient transport to tertiary care center.

- **Children >20 kg:** 4 mL/kg per hour for the first 10 kg + 2 mL/kg per hour for kg 11-20 + 1 mL/kg per hour for each kg above 20 kg.

  Example: For a 28-kg child, estimated maintenance fluid rate
  = (4 mL/kg per hour × 10 kg)
    + (2 mL/kg per hour × 10 kg)
    + (1 mL/kg per hour × 8 kg)
  = 40 mL per hour + 20 mL per hour
    + 8 mL per hour
  = 68 mL per hour

After initial stabilization, adjust the rate and composition of intravenous fluids based on the patient's clinical condition and state of hydration. In general, provide a continuous infusion of a dextrose-containing solution for infants. Avoid hypotonic solutions in critically ill children; for most patients use isotonic fluid such as normal saline (0.9% NaCl) or lactated Ringer's solution with or without dextrose, based on the child's clinical status.

Pediatric Resuscitation Supplies
Based on Color-Coded Resuscitation Tape

Equipment	GRAY* 3-5 kg	PINK Small Infant 6-7 kg	RED Infant 8-9 kg	PURPLE Toddler 10-11 kg	YELLOW Small Child 12-14 kg	WHITE Child 15-18 kg	BLUE Child 19-23 kg	ORANGE Large Child 24-29 kg	GREEN Adult 30-36 kg
Resuscitation bag		Infant/child	Infant/child	Child	Child	Child	Child	Child	Adult
Oxygen mask (NRB)		Pediatric	Pediatric	Pediatric	Pediatric	Pediatric	Pediatric	Pediatric	Pediatric/adult
Oral airway (mm)		50	50	60	60	60	70	80	80
Laryngoscope blade (size)		1 Straight	1 Straight	1 Straight	2 Straight	2 Straight	2 Straight or curved	2 Straight or curved	3 Straight or curved
ET tube (mm)[†]		3.5 Uncuffed 3.0 Cuffed	3.5 Uncuffed 3.0 Cuffed	4.0 Uncuffed 3.5 Cuffed	4.5 Uncuffed 4.0 Cuffed	5.0 Uncuffed 4.5 Cuffed	5.5 Uncuffed 5.0 Cuffed	6.0 Cuffed	6.5 Cuffed
ET tube insertion length (cm)	3 kg 9-9.5 4 kg 9.5-10 5 kg 10-10.5	10.5-11	10.5-11	11-12	13.5	14-15	16.5	17-18	18.5-19.5
Suction catheter (F)		8	8	10	10	10	10	10	10-12
BP cuff	Neonatal #5/infant	Infant/child	Infant/child	Child	Child	Child	Child	Child	Small adult
IV catheter (ga)		22-24	22-24	20-24	18-22	18-22	18-20	18-20	16-20
IO (ga)		18/15	18/15	15	15	15	15	15	15
NG tube (F)		5-8	5-8	8-10	10	10	12-14	14-18	16-18
Urinary catheter (F)	5	8	8	8-10	10	10-12	10-12	12	12
Chest tube (F)		10-12	10-12	16-20	20-24	20-24	24-32	28-32	32-38

Abbreviations: BP, blood pressure; ET, endotracheal; F, French; IO, intraosseous; IV, intravenous; NG, nasogastric; NRB, nonrebreathing.

*For Gray column, use Pink or Red equipment sizes if no size is listed.

[†]Per *2005 AHA Guidelines*, in the hospital cuffed or uncuffed tubes may be used (see below for sizing of cuffed tubes).

Adapted from *Broselow™ Pediatric Emergency Tape*. Distributed by Armstrong Medical Industries, Lincolnshire, IL. 2007 Vital Signs, Inc.

Estimating Endotracheal Tube Size and Depth of Insertion

Tube Size

Several formulas, such as the ones below, allow estimation of proper endotracheal tube size (internal diameter [i.d.]) for children 2 to 10 years of age, based on the child's age:

Uncuffed endotracheal tube size (mm i.d.) = (age in years/4) + 4

During preparation for intubation, providers also should have ready at the bedside uncuffed endotracheal tubes 0.5 mm smaller and larger than that estimated from the above formula.

The formula for estimation of a cuffed endotracheal tube size is as follows:

Cuffed endotracheal tube size (mm i.d.) = (age in years/4) + 3.5

Typical cuffed inflation pressure should be <20 to 25 cm H_2O.

Depth of Insertion

The formula for estimation of depth of insertion (measured at the lip) can be estimated from the child's age or the tube size.

Depth of insertion (cm) for children >2 years of age = (age in years/2) + 12

or

Depth of insertion = tube i.d. (mm) × 3

Confirm placement with both clinical assessment (eg, breath sounds, chest expansion) and device (eg, exhaled CO_2 detector). Watch for marker on endotracheal tube at vocal cords.

Administration Notes

Peripheral intravenous (IV):	Resuscitation drugs administered via peripheral IV catheter should be followed by a bolus of at least 5 mL NS to move drug into central circulation.
Intraosseous (IO):	Drugs that can be administered by IV route can be administered by IO route. They should be followed by a bolus of at least 5 mL NS to move drug into central circulation.
Endotracheal:	IV/IO administration is preferred because it provides more reliable drug delivery and pharmacologic effect. Drugs that can be administered by endotracheal route are noted in the table below. Optimal endotracheal doses have not yet been established. Doses given by endotracheal route should generally be higher than standard IV doses. For infants and children, dilute the medication with NS to a volume of 3 to 5 mL, instill in the endotracheal tube, and follow with flush of 3 to 5 mL. Provide 5 positive-pressure breaths after medication is instilled.
Formula for verification of dose and continuous infusion rate:	Infusion rate (mL/h) = $\dfrac{\text{Weight (kg)} \times \text{dose (mcg/kg per minute)} \times 60 \text{ min/h}}{\text{Concentration (mcg/mL)}}$

Adenosine

Indications
Drug of choice for treatment of symptomatic SVT.

Precautions
- Very short half-life.
- Limited adult data suggest need to reduce dose in patients taking carbamazepine and dipyridamole.
- Less effective (larger doses may be required) in patients taking theophylline or caffeine.

IV/IO Administration
- First dose
  - 0.1 mg/kg IV/IO *rapid* push.
  - Maximum dose: 6 mg.
- Second dose
  - 0.2 mg/kg IV/IO *rapid* push.
  - Maximum dose: 12 mg.
- Follow immediately with 5 to 10 mL NS flush.
- Continuous ECG monitoring.

Injection Technique
- Record rhythm strip during administration.
- Draw up adenosine dose in one syringe and flush in another. Attach both syringes to the same or immediately adjacent IV injection ports nearest patient, with adenosine closest to patient.
- Clamp IV tubing above injection port.
- Push IV adenosine as *quickly* as possible (1 to 3 seconds).
- While maintaining pressure on adenosine plunger, push NS flush *as rapidly as possible* after adenosine.
- Unclamp IV tubing.

Drug/Therapy	Indications/Precautions	Pediatric Dosage
Albuterol Nebulized solution: 0.5% (5 mg/mL) Prediluted nebulized solution: 0.63 mg/3 mL NS, 1.25 mg/3 mL NS, 2.5 mg/3 mL NS (0.083%) MDI: 90 mcg/puff	**Indications** Bronchodilator, β_2-adrenergic agent • Asthma. • Anaphylaxis (bronchospasm). • Hyperkalemia.	**For Asthma, Anaphylaxis (Mild to Moderate), Hyperkalemia** • **MDI (every 20 minutes)** — 4 to 8 puffs (inhalation) PRN with spacer. • **Nebulizer (every 20 minutes)** — Weight <20 kg: 2.5 mg/dose (inhalation). — Weight >20 kg: 5 mg/dose (inhalation). **For Asthma, Anaphylaxis (Severe)** • **Continuous nebulizer** — 0.5 mg/kg per hour continuous inhalation (maximum dose 20 mg/h). • **MDI (recommended if intubated)** — 4 to 8 puffs (inhalation) via endotracheal tube every 20 minutes PRN or with spacer if not intubated.

Alprostadil (PGE$_1$)
(see Prostaglandin E$_1$)

Amiodarone

Indications

Can be used for treatment of atrial and ventricular arrhythmias in children, particularly ectopic atrial tachycardia, junctional ectopic tachycardia, and ventricular tachycardia/ventricular fibrillation.

Precautions

- May produce hypotension. May prolong QT interval and increase propensity for polymorphic ventricular arrhythmias. Therefore, routine administration in combination with procainamide is not recommended without expert consultation.
- Use with caution if hepatic failure is present.
- Terminal elimination is extremely long (elimination half-life with long-term oral dosing is up to 40 days).

For Refractory VF, Pulseless VT

- 5 mg/kg IV/IO bolus; can repeat the 5 mg/kg IV/IO bolus up to total dose of 15 mg/kg (2.2 g in adolescents) IV per 24 hours.
- Maximum single dose: 300 mg.

For Perfusing Supraventricular and Ventricular Arrhythmias

Loading dose: 5 mg/kg IV/IO over 20 to 60 minutes (maximum single dose: 300 mg). Can repeat to maximum of 15 mg/kg (2.2 g in adolescents) per day IV.

Drug/Therapy	Indications/Precautions	Pediatric Dosage

Atropine Sulfate
 	
Can be given by endotracheal tube
	Indications
	• Symptomatic bradycardia (usually secondary to vagal stimulation).
	• Toxins/overdose (organophosphate and carbamate poisoning).
	• Rapid sequence intubation (RSI): ie, age <1 year, age 1 to 5 years receiving succinylcholine, age >5 years receiving second dose of succinylcholine.
	
	Precautions
	• Contraindicated in angle-closure glaucoma, tachyarrhythmias, and thyrotoxicosis.
	• Drug blocks bradycardic response to hypoxia. Monitor with pulse oximetry.
		Symptomatic Bradycardia
		• **IV/IO:** 0.02 mg/kg.
		  — Maximum single dose: 0.5 mg.
		  — May repeat dose once in 3 to 5 minutes.
		  — Maximum total dose for child: 1 mg; for adolescent: 3 mg.
		  — Larger doses may be needed for organophosphate poisoning.
		• **Endotracheal:** 0.04 to 0.06 mg/kg.
		
		Toxins/Overdose (Organophosphate and Carbamate Poisoning)
		• <12 years: 0.05 mg/kg IV/IO initially; then repeated and doubling the dose every 5 minutes until muscarinic symptoms reverse.
		• ≥12 years: 1 mg IV/IO initially; then repeated and doubling the dose every 5 minutes until muscarinic symptoms reverse.
		
		RSI
		• **IV/IO:** 0.01 to 0.02 mg/kg (maximum dose: 0.5 mg).
		• **IM:** 0.02 mg/kg.

Calcium Chloride

10% = 100 mg/mL = 27.2 mg/mL elemental calcium

Indications
- Treatment of documented or suspected conditions
  - Hypocalcemia.
  - Hyperkalemia.
- Consider for treatment of
  - Hypermagnesemia.
  - Calcium channel blocker overdose.

Precautions
- Do not use routinely during resuscitation (may contribute to cellular injury).
- Not recommended for routine treatment of asystole or PEA.
- Rapid IV administration may cause hypotension, bradycardia, or asystole (particularly if patient is receiving digoxin).
- Do not mix with or infuse immediately before or after sodium bicarbonate without intervening flush.

IV/IO Administration
- 20 mg/kg (0.2 mL/kg) slow IV/IO push.
- May repeat if documented or suspected clinical indication persists (eg, toxicologic problem).
- Central venous administration preferred if available.

Drug/Therapy	Indications/Precautions	Pediatric Dosage

Calcium Gluconate
 	
10% = 100 mg/mL = 9 mg/mL elemental calcium
	Indications
	• Treatment of documented or suspected conditions
	  — Hypocalcemia.
	  — Hyperkalemia.
	• Consider for treatment of
	  — Hypermagnesemia.
	  — Calcium channel blocker overdose.
	
	Precautions
	• Do not use routinely during resuscitation (may contribute to cellular injury).
	• Not recommended for routine treatment of asystole or PEA.
	• Rapid IV administration may cause hypotension, bradycardia, or asystole (particularly if patient is receiving digoxin).
	• Do not mix with or infuse immediately before or after sodium bicarbonate without intervening flush.
		IV/IO Administration
		• 60 mg/kg (0.6 mL/kg) slow IV/IO push.
		• May repeat if documented or suspected clinical indication persists (eg, toxicologic problem).
		• Central venous administration preferred if available.

Corticosteroids

Precautions
May cause hypertension, hyperglycemia, and increased risk of gastric bleeding.

Dexamethasone

Indications
- Croup.
- Asthma.

Dexamethasone
For Croup
0.6 mg/kg PO/IM/IV × 1 dose (maximum dose: 16 mg).

For Asthma
0.6 mg/kg PO/IM/IV every 24 hours (maximum dose: 16 mg).

Hydrocortisone

Indications
Treatment of adrenal insufficiency (may be associated with septic shock).

Hydrocortisone
Adrenal Insufficiency
2 mg/kg IV/IO bolus (maximum dose: 100 mg).

Methylprednisolone

Indications
- Asthma (status asthmaticus).
- Anaphylactic shock.

Methylprednisolone
Use sodium succinate salt.

Status Asthmaticus, Anaphylactic Shock
- Load: 2 mg/kg IV/IO/IM (maximum: 60 mg).
- Maintenance: 0.5 mg/kg IV every 6 hours or 1 mg/kg every 12 hours up to 120 mg/day.

Drug/Therapy	Indications/Precautions	Pediatric Dosage
Dobutamine	**Indications** Treatment of shock associated with high systemic vascular resistance (eg, congestive heart failure or cardiogenic shock). Ensure adequate intravascular volume. **Precautions** • May produce or exacerbate hypotension. • May produce tachyarrhythmias. • Do not mix with sodium bicarbonate. • Extravasation may cause tissue injury.	**Continuous IV/IO Infusion** Titrate to desired effect. Typical infusion dose: 2 to 20 mcg/kg per minute.

Dopamine

Indications

Treatment of shock with adequate intravascular volume and stable rhythm.

Precautions

- High infusion rates (>20 mcg/kg per minute) may cause splanchnic vasoconstriction, ischemia.
- May produce tachyarrhythmias.
- Do not mix with sodium bicarbonate.
- Extravasation may cause tissue injury.
- May affect thyroid function.

Continuous IV/IO Infusion

Titrate to desired effect. Typical infusion dose: 2 to 20 mcg/kg per minute.

Note: If infusion dose >20 mcg/kg per minute is required, consider using alternative adrenergic agent (eg, epinephrine/norepinephrine).

Drug/Therapy	Indications/Precautions	Pediatric Dosage

Epinephrine
 	
Standard: 1:10 000 or 0.1 mg/mL
 	
High: 1:1000 or 1 mg/mL
 	
Can be given via endotracheal tube
	Indications
	• Bolus IV therapy
	  — Treatment of pulseless arrest.
	  — Treatment of symptomatic bradycardia unresponsive to O_2 and ventilation.
	• Continuous IV infusion
	  — Shock (poor perfusion) or hypotension in patient with adequate intravascular volume and stable rhythm.
	  — Clinically significant bradycardia.
	  — β-Blocker or calcium channel blocker overdose.
	  — Pulseless arrest when bolus therapy fails.
	• IM bolus therapy
	  — Anaphylaxis.
	  — Severe status asthmaticus.
		Pulseless Arrest
		• **IV/IO dose:** 0.01 mg/kg (0.1 mL/kg of 1:10 000 standard concentration). Administer every 3 to 5 minutes during arrest (maximum dose: 1 mg).
		• **All endotracheal doses:** 0.1 mg/kg (0.1 mL/kg of 1:1000 high concentration).
		  — Administer every 3 to 5 minutes of arrest until IV/IO access achieved; then begin with first IV dose.
		
		Symptomatic Bradycardia
		• **All IV/IO doses:** 0.01 mg/kg (0.1 mL/kg of 1:10 000 standard concentration).
		• **All endotracheal doses:** 0.1 mg/kg (0.1 mL/kg of 1:1000 high concentration).

(continued)   ↓   ↓

Epinephrine
(continued)

Precautions
- May produce tachyarrhythmias.
- High-dose infusions may produce vasoconstriction or may compromise perfusion; low doses may decrease renal and splanchnic blood flow.
- Do not mix with sodium bicarbonate.
- Correct hypoxemia.
- Contraindicated in treatment of VT secondary to cocaine (may be considered if VF develops).

Continuous IV/IO Infusion
Once tubing is primed, titrate to response. Typical initial infusion: 0.1 to 1 mcg/kg per minute. Higher doses may be effective.

Anaphylaxis/Severe Status Asthmaticus
- IM dose: 0.01 mg/kg (0.01 mL/kg of 1:1000 high concentration).
- Maximum single dose: 0.3 mg.
- Repeat as needed.

Drug/Therapy	Indications/Precautions	Pediatric Dosage
Etomidate	**Indications** • Ultrashort-acting nonbarbiturate, non-benzodiazepine sedative-hypnotic agent with no analgesic properties. • Produces rapid sedation with minimal cardiovascular or respiratory depression. • Sedative of choice for hypotensive patients. • Decreases ICP, cerebral blood flow, and cerebral basal metabolic rate. **Precautions** • May suppress cortisol production after a single dose. Consider administration of stress dose hydrocortisone (2 mg/kg; maximum dose 100 mg). • Avoid routine use in septic shock. • May also cause myoclonic activity (coughing, hiccups) and may exacerbate focal seizure disorders. • Relative contraindications include known adrenal insufficiency or history of focal seizure disorder.	**For Rapid Sedation** • IV/IO dose of 0.2 to 0.4 mg/kg infused over 30 to 60 seconds will produce rapid sedation that lasts 10 to 15 minutes. • Maximum dose: 20 mg.

Glucose

Indications
Treatment of hypoglycemia (documented or strongly suspected).

Precautions
- Use bedside glucose test to confirm hypoglycemia; hyperglycemia may worsen neurologic outcome of cardiopulmonary arrest or trauma; do not administer routinely during resuscitation
- Maximum concentration for newborn administration: 12.5% (0.125 g/mL).

IV/IO Infusion
- 0.5 to 1 g/kg (maximum recommended IV/IO concentration: 25%; can prepare by mixing 50% dextrose 1:1 with sterile water).
  - **50%** dextrose (0.5 g/mL); give 1 to 2 mL/kg.
  - **25%** dextrose (0.25 g/mL); give 2 to 4 mL/kg.
  - **10%** dextrose (0.1 g/mL); give 5 to 10 mL/kg.
  - **5%** dextrose (0.05 g/mL); give 10 to 20 mL/kg if volume tolerated.

Ipratropium Bromide

Indications
Anticholinergic and bronchodilator used for treatment of asthma.

Precautions
May cause pupil dilation if it enters eyes.

Inhalation Dose
250 to 500 mcg (by nebulizer, MDI) every 20 minutes × 3 doses.

Drug/Therapy	Indications/Precautions	Pediatric Dosage

Lidocaine

Can be given via endotracheal tube

Indications
- Bolus therapy
  - VF/pulseless VT.
  - Wide-complex tachycardia (with pulses).
- RSI: May decrease ICP response during laryngoscopy.

Precautions/Contraindications
- High plasma concentration may cause myocardial and circulatory depression, possible CNS symptoms (eg, seizures).
- Reduce infusion dose if severe CHF or low cardiac output is compromising hepatic and renal blood flow.
- Contraindicated for bradycardia with wide-complex ventricular escape beats.

VF/Pulseless VT, Wide-Complex Tachycardia (With Pulses)
- **IV/IO**
  - Initial: 1 mg/kg IV/IO loading dose.
  - Maintenance: 20 to 50 mcg/kg per minute IV/IO infusion (repeat bolus dose if infusion initiated >15 minutes after initial bolus therapy).
- **Endotracheal:** 2 to 3 mg/kg.

RSI
1 to 2 mg/kg IV/IO.

Magnesium Sulfate

50% = 500 mg/mL

Indications
- Torsades de pointes or suspected hypomagnesemia.
- Status asthmaticus not responsive to β-adrenergic drugs.

Precautions/Contraindications
- Contraindicated in renal failure.
- Possible hypotension and bradycardia with rapid bolus.

Pulseless VT With Torsades
25 to 50 mg/kg IV/IO bolus (maximum dose: 2 g).

Torsades (With Pulses), Hypomagnesemia
25 to 50 mg/kg IV/IO (maximum dose: 2 g) over 10 to 20 minutes.

Status Asthmaticus
25 to 50 mg/kg IV/IO (maximum dose: 2 g) over 15 to 30 minutes.

Milrinone

Indications
Cardiogenic shock or heart failure marked by low contractility, high vascular resistance, or both.

Precautions/Contraindications
- May cause hypotension.
- May cause arrhythmias.
- Eliminated by renal excretion; use with caution in patients with renal insufficiency.
- Avoid in patients with ventricular outflow tract obstruction.

Loading Dose
50 mcg/kg. Administer over 10 to 60 minutes. Monitor for hypotension.

IV Infusion
Maintenance dose (continuous IV infusion): 0.25 to 0.75 mcg/kg per minute.

Drug/Therapy	Indications/Precautions	Pediatric Dosage
Naloxone Can be given IV/IO/IM/subcutaneously Can be given via endotracheal tube; other routes preferred	**Indications** To reverse effects of narcotic toxicity: respiratory depression, hypotension, and hypoperfusion. **Precautions** • Half-life of naloxone often shorter than half-life of narcotic; repeated dosing is often required. • Administration to infants of addicted mothers may precipitate seizures or other withdrawal symptoms. • Assist ventilation before administration to avoid sympathetic stimulation. • May reverse effects of analgesics; consider administration of nonopioid analgesics for treatment of pain.	**Bolus IV/IO/IM/ Subcutaneous Dose** For *total* reversal of narcotic effects, give 0.1 mg/kg every 2 minutes PRN (maximum dose: 2 mg). *Note:* If total reversal is not required (eg, respiratory depression), smaller doses (0.001 to 0.005 mg/kg [1 to 5 mcg/kg]) may be used. Titrate to effect. **Continuous IV/IO Infusion** 0.002 to 0.16 mg/kg (2 to 160 mcg/kg) per hour IV/IO infusion.
Nitroglycerin	**Indications** • Heart failure (especially associated with myocardial ischemia). • Hypertensive emergency. • Pulmonary hypertension.	**Dose (Continuous IV Infusion)** • Initial dose: 0.25 to 0.5 mcg/kg per minute. • Titrate by 1 mcg/kg per minute every 15 to 20 minutes as tolerated.

(continued)

Nitroglycerin
(continued)

Precautions
May cause hypotension, especially in hypovolemic patients.

- Typical dose range: 1 to 5 mcg/kg per minute (maximum dose: 10 mcg/kg per minute).
- In adolescents, start with 5 to 10 mcg *per minute* (this dose is *not* per kilogram per minute), and increase to maximum of 200 mcg *per minute*.

Nitroprusside
(Sodium nitroprusside)

Mix in D_5W

Vasodilator that reduces tone in all vascular beds.

Indications
- Shock or low cardiac output states (cardiogenic shock) characterized by high vascular resistance.
- Severe hypertension.

Precautions
- May cause hypotension, particularly with hypovolemia.
- Metabolized by endothelial cells to cyanide, then metabolized in liver to thiocyanate and excreted by kidneys. Thiocyanate and cyanide toxicity may result if administered at high rates or with decreased hepatic or renal function. Monitor thiocyanate levels in patients receiving prolonged infusion, particularly if rate >2 mcg/kg per minute.
- Signs of thiocyanate toxicity include seizures, nausea, vomiting, metabolic acidosis, and abdominal cramps.

IV/IO Infusion
- 0.3 to 1 mcg/kg per minute initially; then titrate up to 8 mcg/kg per minute as needed.
- Light sensitive; cover drug reservoir with opaque material, or use specialized administration set.
- Typically change solution every 24 hours.

Drug/Therapy	Indications/Precautions	Pediatric Dosage
Norepinephrine	Sympathetic neurotransmitter with inotropic effects. Activates myocardial β-adrenergic receptors and vascular α-adrenergic receptors. **Indications** Treatment of shock and hypotension characterized by low systemic vascular resistance and unresponsive to fluid resuscitation. **Precautions** • May produce hypertension, organ ischemia, and arrhythmias. Extravasation may cause tissue necrosis (treat with phentolamine). • Do not administer in same IV tubing with alkaline solutions.	**IV Administration (Only Route)** Begin at rates of 0.1 to 2 mcg/kg per minute; adjust infusion rate to achieve desired change in blood pressure and systemic perfusion.
Oxygen	**Indications** • Should be administered during stabilization of all seriously ill or injured patients with respiratory insufficiency, shock, or trauma, even if oxyhemoglobin saturation is normal. • May monitor pulse oximetry to evaluate oxygenation and titrate therapy once child has adequate perfusion.	• Administer in highest possible concentration during initial evaluation and stabilization. • A nonrebreathing mask with reservoir delivers 95% oxygen with flow rate of 10 to 15 L/min. • After cardiac arrest, maintain oxyhemoglobin saturation 94% to 99% (or as appropriate to the patient's condition) to minimize risk of oxidative injury.

Procainamide

Indications
SVT, atrial flutter, VT (with pulses).

Precautions
- Seek expert consultation when using this agent.
- Routine use in combination with amiodarone (or other drugs that prolong QT interval) is not recommended without expert consultation.
- Risk of hypotension and negative inotropic effects increases with rapid administration; not appropriate agent for VF/pulseless VT.
- Reduce dose for patients with poor renal or cardiac function.

Loading Dose
15 mg/kg IV/IO over 30 to 60 minutes.

Prostaglandin E₁ (PGE₁)
(Alprostadil)

Indications
To maintain patency of ductus arteriosus in newborns with cyanotic congenital heart disease and ductal-dependent pulmonary or systemic blood flow.

Precautions
- May produce vasodilation, hypotension, apnea, hyperpyrexia, agitation, seizures.
- May produce hypoglycemia, hypocalcemia.

IV/IO Administration
- **Initial:** 0.05 to 0.1 mcg/kg per minute IV/IO infusion.
- **Maintenance:** 0.01 to 0.05 mcg/kg per minute IV/IO infusion.

Drug/Therapy	Indications/Precautions	Pediatric Dosage
Sodium Bicarbonate 8.4%: 1 mEq/mL in 10- or 50-mL syringe 4.2%: 0.5 mEq/mL in 10-mL syringe	**Indications** • Treatment of severe metabolic acidosis (documented or following prolonged arrest) unresponsive to ventilation and oxygenation. • Treatment of the following: — Hyperkalemia. — Sodium channel blocker toxicity, such as tricyclic antidepressants (after support of adequate airway and ventilation). **Precautions** • Routine administration is not recommended in cardiac arrest. • Infuse slowly. • Buffering action will produce carbon dioxide, so ventilation must be adequate. • Do not mix with any resuscitation drugs. Flush IV tubing with NS before and after drug administration. • Infiltration will cause tissue irritation.	**IV/IO Administration** **Metabolic Acidosis (Severe), Hyperkalemia** • IV/IO: 1 mEq/kg *slow* bolus. • 4.2% concentration recommended for use in infants <1 month of age. **Sodium Channel Blocker Overdose (eg, Tricyclic Antidepressant)** 1 to 2 mEq/kg IV/IO bolus until serum pH is >7.45 (7.50 to 7.55 for severe poisoning) followed by IV/IO infusion of 150 mEq $NaHCO_3$/L solution to maintain alkalosis.

Vasopressin

Indications
Catecholamine-resistant hypotension.

Precautions
Use with caution in patients with renal insufficiency or hyponatremia/free water overload.

Hypotension (continuous IV infusion): 0.0002 to 0.002 unit/kg per minute (0.2 to 2 milliunits/kg per minute).